6.00

The
Art of
Seeing

The Art of Seeing

by Aldous Huxley
Foreword by
Laura Huxley

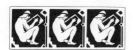

Creative Arts Book Company

Contents

Foreword
by Laura Huxley

I am delighted at the good news: one does not need to be a clairvoyant to predict that the republication of The Art of Seeing *is an enriching event.*

Although published forty years ago this book is timely in many ways—first of all we certainly need to see more clearly! Secondly, it is encouraging to be reminded that it is our response to adverse events that gives quality to our life. The Art of Seeing *was Aldous' response to the fact that his sight was rapidly failing and that, in a matter of a short time, he would be blind. With an open mind he studied the Bates Method which, still now but especially in 1939, was unaccepted by the orthodox ophthalmologist. His eyesight and that of thousands of others was improved, even saved.*

Besides the disciplines from the East, the movement for the development of human potentialities has ushered in many unconventional methods: those of F.M. Alexander (which Aldous practiced years ago), of Reich and Bioenergetics, of Rolf, Feldenkrais and others. These methods and The Art of Seeing *recognize that, in the human condition, mind and body are inextricably connected.* The Art of Seeing *was a forerunner of these body-mind techniques which dovetail and enhance each other.*

Congratulations to the publishers on their own clear vision through which many people will see better.

Laura Huxley
Hollywood, California

Preface

At sixteen I had a violent attack of *keratitis punctata*, which left me (after eighteen months of near-blindness, during which I had to depend on Braille for my reading and a guide for my walking) with one eye just capable of light perception, and the other with enough vision to permit of my detecting the two-hundred foot letter on the Snellen chart at ten feet. My inability to see was mainly due to the presence of opacities in the cornea; but this condition was complicated by hyperopia and astigmatism. For the first few years my doctors advised me to do my reading with the aid of a powerful hand magnifying glass. But later on I was promoted to spectacles. With the aid of these I was able to recognize the seventy-foot line at ten feet and to read tolerably well—provided always that I kept my better pupil dilated with atropine, so that I might see round a particularly heavy patch of opacity at the center of the cornea. True, a measure of strain and fatigue was always present, and there were occasions when I was overcome by the sense of complete physical and mental exhaustion which only eye-strain can produce. Still, I was grateful to be able to see as well as I could.

Things went on in this way until the year 1939, when in spite of greatly strengthened glasses I found the task of reading increasingly difficult and fatiguing. There could be no doubt of it: my capacity to see was steadily and quite rapidly failing. But just as I was wondering apprehensively what on earth I should do, if reading were to become impossible, I happened to hear of a method of visual re-education and of a teacher who was said to make use of this method with conspicuous success. Education sounded harmless enough and, since optical glass was no longer doing me any good, I decided to take the plunge. Within a couple of months I was reading without spectacles and, what was better still, without strain and fatigue. The chronic tensions and the occasional spells of complete exhaustion were things of the past. Moreover, there were definite signs that the opacity in the cornea, which had remained unchanged for upwards of twenty-five years, was beginning to clear up. At the present time, my vision, though very far from normal, is about twice as good as it used to be when I wore spectacles, and before I had learned the art of seeing; and the opacity has cleared sufficiently to permit the worse eye, which for years could do no more than distinguish light from darkness, to recognize the ten-foot line on the chart at one foot.

It is, first of all, to repay a debt of gratitude that I have written this little book—gratitude to the pioneer of visual education, the late Dr. W.H. Bates, and to his disciple, Mrs. Margaret D. Corbett, to whose skill as a teacher I owe the improvement in my own vision.

A number of other books on visual education have been published—notably Dr. Bates' own, *Perfect Sight Without Glasses* (New York, 1920), Mrs. Corbetts' *How to Improve Your Eyes* (Los Angeles, 1938) and *The Improvement of Sight by Natural Methods*, by C.S. Price, M.B.E., D.O. (London, 1934). All have their merits; but in none (of those, at least, that I have read) has an attempt been made to do what I have tried to do in the present volume; namely, to correlate the methods of visual education with the findings of modern psychology and critical philosophy. My purpose in making this correlaton is to demonstrate the essential reasonableness of a method, which turns out to be nothing more nor less than the practical application to the problems of vision of certain theoretical principles universally accepted as true.

Why, it may be asked, have orthodox ophthalmologists failed to make these applications of universally accepted principles? The answer is clear. Ever since ophthalmology became a science, its practitioners have been obsessively preoccupied with only one aspect of the total, complex process of seeing—the physiological. They have paid attention exclusively to eyes, not at all to the mind which makes use of the eyes to see with. I have been treated by men of the highest eminence in their profession; but never once did they so much as faintly hint that there might be a mental side to vision, or that there might be wrong ways of using the eyes and mind as well as right ways, unnatural and abnormal modes of visual functioning as well as natural and normal ones. After checking the acute infection in my eyes, which they did with the greatest skill, they gave me some artificial lenses and let me go. Whether I used my mind and be-spectacled eyes well or badly, and what might be the effect upon my vision of improper use, were to them, as to practically all other orthodox ophthalmologists, matters of perfect indifference. To Dr. Bates, on the contrary, these things were not matters of indifference; and because they were not, he worked out, through long years of experiment and clinical practice, his peculiar method of visual education. That this method was essentially sound is proved by its efficacy. My own case is in no way unique; thousands of other sufferers from defects of vision have benefited by following the simple rules of that Art of Seeing, which we owe to Bates and his followers. To make this Art more widely known is the final purpose of the present volume.

Chapter 1

Medicine and Defective Vision

Medicus curat, natura sanat—the doctor treats, nature heals. The old aphorism sums up the whole scope and purpose of medicine, which is to provide sick organisms with the internal and external conditions most favorable to the exercise of their own self-regulative and restorative powers. If there were no *vis medicatrix naturae,* no natural healing powers, medicine would be helpless, and every small derangement would either kill outright or settle down into chronic disease.

When conditions are favorable sick organisms tend to recover through their own inherent powers of self-healing. If they do not recover it means either that the case is hopeless, or that the conditions are not favorable—in other words, that the medical treatment being applied is failing to achieve what an adequate treatment ought to achieve.

Ordinary Treatment of
Defective Sight

In the light of these general principles let us consider the current medical treatment of defects of vision. In the great majority of cases the only treatment consists in fitting the patient with artificial lenses designed to correct the particular error of refraction which is held to be responsible for the defect. *Medicus curat;* and in most cases the patient is rewarded by an immediate improvement in vision. But in the meanwhile, what about Nature and her healing process? Do glasses eliminate the causes of defective vision? Do the organs of sight tend to revert to normal functioning as the result of the treatment with artificial lenses? The answer to these questions is, No. Artificial lenses neutralize the symptoms, but do not get rid of the causes of defective vision. And so far from improving, eyes fitted with these devices tend to grow progressively weaker and to require progressively stronger lenses for the correction of their symptoms. In a word, *medicus curat, natura non sanat.* From this we can draw one of two conclusions: either defects in the organs of seeing are incurable, and can only be palliated by mechanical neutralizations of symptoms; or else something is radically wrong with the current methods of treatment.

Orthodox opinion accepts the first and more pessimistic alternative, and insists that the mechanical palliation of symptoms is the only kind of treatment to which defective organs of vision will respond. (I am leaving out of account all cases of more or less acute disease of the eyes, which are treated by surgery and medication, and confining myself to those much more commonplace visual defects now treated by means of lenses.)

Cure or Palliation of Symptoms?

If orthodox opinion is right—if the organs of vision are incapable of curing themselves, and if their defects can only be palliated by mechanical devices—then the eyes must be totally different in kind from other parts of the body. Given favorable conditions, all other organs tend to free themselves from their defects. Not so the eyes. When they show symptoms of weakness, it is foolish, according to orthodox theory, to make any serious effort to get rid of the causes of those symptoms: it is a waste of time even to try to discover a treatment which will assist nature in accomplishing its normal task of healing. Defective eyes are, *ex hypothesi,* practically incurable; they lack the *vis medicatrix naturae.* The only thing that ophthalmo-logical science can do for them is to provide them with the purely mechanical means for neutralizing their symptoms. The only qualifi-cations to this strange theory come from those who have made it their business to look into external conditions of seeing. Here, for example, are some relevant remarks taken from the book *Seeing and Human Welfare* by Dr. Matthew Luckiesh, Director of the General Electric Company's Lighting Research Laboratory. Eyeglasses (those "valuable crutches," as Dr. Luckiesh calls them) "counteract effects of heredity, age and *abuse;* they do not deal with causes." "Suppose that crippled eyes could be transformed into crippled legs. What a heart-rending parade we would witness on a busy street! Nearly every other person would go limping by. Many would be on crutches and some on wheel chairs. How many of these defects of the eye are due to poor conditions for seeing, that is, to indifference towards seeing? Statis-tics are not available, but a knowledge of seeing and its requirements indicates that most of them are preventable and most of the remain-der can be improved or arrested by adequate and proper conditions." And again, "even the refractive defects and other abnormalities of eyes induced by abuses are not necessarily permanent. When we become ill, Nature does her part, if we do ours, towards getting well. Eyes have various recuperative powers, at least to some degree. Reducing their abuse by improving seeing conditions is always help-ful, and there are many cases on record where great improvement has followed on this procedure. Indeed, without correction of the abuse, the disorder generally becomes progressively worse." These are encouraging words that leave us with the hope that we are to be given a description of some new and genuinely aetiological treatment of visual defects, to take the place of the purely symptomatic treatment at present in vogue. But this hope is only imperfectly fulfilled. "Poor lighting," Dr. Luckiesh goes on, "is the most important and universal cause of eye strain, often leading to progressive defects and dis-orders." His whole book is an elaboration of this theme. Let me hasten to add that, within its limitations, it is an admirable book. To those suffering from defects of vision the importance of good lighting is very great indeed; and one can only be grateful to Dr. Luckiesh for his scientific clarification of the meaning "good lighting" in terms of standard, measurable entities such as foot-candles. One's only complaint is that foot-candles are not enough. In treating other parts of the organism doctors are not content to ameliorate merely the external conditions of functioning; they also seek to improve the internal conditions, to work directly on the physiological environment of the sick organ as well as on the physical environment outside the body. Thus when legs are crippled, doctors refuse to let their patients rely indefinitely on crutches. Nor do they consider that the laying down of rules for avoiding accidents constitutes sufficient treatment for the condition of being crippled. On the contrary, they regard the use of crutches as merely a palliative and temporary expedient, and while paying attention to external conditions, they also do their best to improve the internal conditions of the defective part, so that nature may be helped to do its work of healing. Some of these measures, such as rest, massage, applications of heat and light, make no appeal to the patient's mind, but are aimed directly at the affected organs, their purpose being to relax, to increase circulation and to preserve mobility. Other measures are educational and involve, on the patient's part, a coordination of mind and body. By means of this appeal to the psychological factor, astonishing results are often obtained. A good teacher, using the right technique, can often educate a victim of accident or paralysis into gradual recovery of his lost functions, and through that recovery of function, into the re-establishment of the health and integrity of the defective organ. If such things can be done for crippled legs, why should it not be possible to do something analogous for defective eyes? To this question the orthodox theory provides no answer—merely takes it for granted that the defective eye is incurable and cannot, in spite of its peculiarly intimate relationship with the psyche, be re-educated towards normality by any process of mind-body coordination.

The orthodox theory is, on the face of it, so implausible, so intrinsically unlikely to be true, that one can only be astonished that it should be so generally and so unquestioningly accepted. Nevertheless, such is the force of habit and authority that we all do accept it. At the present time it is rejected only by those who have personal reasons for knowing it to be untrue. I myself happen to be one of these. By the greatest of good fortune I was given the opportunity to discover by personal experience that eyes do not lack the *vis medicatrix naturae*; that the palliation of symptoms is not the only treatment for defective vision, that the function of sight can be re-educated towards normality by appropriate body-mind coordination, and finally that the improvement in functioning is accompanied by an improvement in the condition of the damaged organ. This personal experience has been confirmed by my observation of many others who have gone through the same process of visual education. It is therefore no longer possible for me to accept the currently orthodox theory, with its hopelessly pessimistic practical corollaries.

Chapter 2

*A Method of Visual
Re-Education*

In the early years of the present century Dr. W.H. Bates, a New York oculist, became dissatisfied with the ordinary symptomatic treatment of eyes. Seeking a substitute for artificial lenses, he set himself to discover if there was any way of re-educating defective vision into a condition of normality.

As the result of his work with a large number of patients, he came to the conclusion that the great majority of visual defects were functional and due to faulty habits of use. These faulty habits of use were invariably related, he found, to a condition of strain and tension. As was to be expected from the unitary nature of the human organism, the strain affected both the body and the mind.

Dr. Bates discovered that, by means of appropriate techniques, this condition of strain could be relieved. When it had been relieved—when patients had learned to use their eyes and mind in a relaxed way—vision was improved and refractive errors tended to correct themselves. Practice in the educational techniques served to build up good seeing habits in place of the faulty habits responsible for defective vision, and in many cases function came to be completely and permanently normalized.

Now, it is a well-established physiological principle that improved functioning always tends to result in an improvement in the organic condition of the tissues involved. The eye, Dr. Bates discovered, was no exception to this general rule. When the patient learned to relax his tenseness and acquired proper seeing habits, the *vis medicatrix naturae* was given a chance to operate—with the result that, in many cases, the improvement of functioning was followed by a complete restoration of the health and organic integrity of the diseased eye.

Dr. Bates died in 1931, and up to the time of his death he continued to perfect and develop his methods for the improvement of visual function. Furthermore, during the last years of Dr. Bates' life and since his death, his pupils in various parts of the world have devised a number of valuable new applications of the general principles which he laid down. By means of these techniques large numbers of men, women and children, suffering from visual defects of every kind, have been successfully re-educated into normality or towards normality. For anyone who has studied a selection of these cases, or who has himself undergone the process of visual re-education, it is impossible to doubt that here at last is a method of treating imperfect sight which is not merely symptomatic, but genuinely aetiological—a method which does not confine itself to the mechanical neutralization of defects but aims at the removal of their physiological and psychological causes. And yet, in spite of the long period during which it has been known, in spite of the quality and quantity of the results obtained through its employment by competent instructors, Dr. Bates' technique still remains unrecognized by the medical and optometrical professions. It is, I think, worth while, before going any further, to enumerate and discuss the principal reasons for this, to my mind, deplorable state of things.

Reasons for Orthodox Disapproval

In the first place, the very fact that the method is unrecognized and lies outside the pale of orthodoxy is a sufficient invitation to the petty adventurers and charlatans who hang upon the skirt of society, ever ready and eager to take advantage of human suffering. There exist, scattered about the world, some scores or perhaps hundreds of well-trained and thoroughly conscientious teachers of Dr. Bates' method. But there are also, unfortunately, a number of ignorant and unscrupulous quacks who know little more of the system than its name. The fact is deplorable, but not at all surprising. The number of those who fail to obtain relief from the current symptomatic treatment of visual defect is considerable, and the Bates Method has a high reputation for effectiveness in such cases. Moreover, the technique is unorthodox; therefore no standards of competence are legally imposed upon its teachers. A large potential clientele, a desperate need of help, and no questions asked as to knowledge, character and ability. These are the ideal conditions for the practice of charlatanism. What wonder, then, if certain unscrupulous people have taken advantage of the opportunities thus offered? But because *some* unorthodox practitioners are charlatans, it does not logically follow that *all* must be. I repeat that it does not logically follow; but, alas, as the history of almost any professional group clearly demonstrates, orthodox opinion would always very much like it to follow. That is one of the reasons why, in this particular case, the unwarranted assumption that the whole business is mere quackery is widely accepted, in spite of all evidence to the contrary. The cure for charlatanism is not the suppression of an intrinsically sound method, but proper education for, and control of, its teachers. Proper education and control are equally the cure for that licensed charlatanism among opticians, which has been described and denounced in articles appearing in *The Readers Digest* (1937) and the New York *World-Telegram* (1942).

The second reason for the non-acceptance of the method may be summed up in three words: habit, authority and professionalism. The symptomatic treatment of defective sight has been going on for a long time, has been carried to a high degree of perfection, and, within its limitations, is reasonably successful. If it fails in a certain proportion of cases to provide even adequate palliation of the symptoms, that is nobody's fault, but a condition inherent in the nature of things. For years the highest medical authorities have all asserted this to be the case—and who will venture to question a recognized authority? Certainly not the members of the profession to which the authority belongs. Every guild and trade has its own *esprit de corps*, its private patriotism, which makes it resent all rebellion from within and all competition or criticism from without.

Next there is the matter of vested interest. The manufacture of optical glass is now a considerable industry, and its retail sale a profitable branch of commerce, to which access can be had only by persons who have undertaken a special technical training. That there should be among these licensed persons a strong dislike to any new technique which threatens to make the use of optical glass unnecessary, is only natural. (It is perhaps worth remarking that, even if the value of Dr. Bates' technique were generally recognized, there would be small likelihood of any immediate or considerable decline in the consumption of optical glass. Visual re-education demands from the pupil a certain amount of thought, time and trouble. But thought, time and trouble are precisely what the overwhelming majority of men and women are not prepared to give unless motivated by a passionate desire or an imperious need. Most of those who can get along more or less satisfactorily with the help of mechanical seeing-aids, will continue to do so, even when they know that there exists a system of training which would make it possible for them, not merely to palliate symptoms, but actually get rid of the causes of visual defect. So long as the art of seeing is not taught to children as a part of their normal education, the trade in artificial lenses is not likely to suffer more than a trifling loss by reason of the official recognition of the new technique. Human sloth and inertia will guarantee the opticians at least nine-tenths of their present business.)

Another reason for the orthodox attitude in this matter is of a strictly empirical nature. Oculists and optometrists affirm that they have never witnessed the phenomena of self-regulation and cure described by Bates and his followers. Therefore they conclude that such phenomena never take place. In this syllogism the premises are true, but the conclusion is unsound. It is quite true that oculists and optometrists have never observed such phenomena as are described by Bates and his followers. But this is because they have never had any dealings with patients who had learned to use their organs of vision in a relaxed, unstrained way. So long as the organs of vision are used under a condition of mental and physical tension, the *vis medicatrix naturae* will not manifest itself, and the visual defects will persist, or actually become worse. Oculists and optometrists will observe the phenomena described by Bates as soon as they begin to relieve the strain in their patients' eyes by means of Bates' method of visual education. Because the phenomena cannot occur under the conditions imposed by orthodox practitioners, it does not follow that they will not occur when these conditions are changed, so that the healing powers of the organism are no longer hindered but given free play.

To this empirical reason for rejecting the Batesian technique must be added one more—this time in the realm of theory. In the course of his practice as an oculist, Dr. Bates came to doubt the truth of the currently accepted hypothesis regarding the eye's power of accommodation to near and distant vision. This matter was for long the subject of heated debate, until finally a couple of generations ago orthodox medical opinion decided in favor of the Helmholtz hypothesis, which attributes the eye's power of accommodation to the action of the ciliary muscle upon the lens. Working with cases of defective vision, Dr. Bates observed a number of facts which the Helmholtz theory seemed powerless to explain. After numerous experiments on animals and human beings, he came to the conclusion that the principal factor in accommodation was not the lens, but the extrinsic muscles of the eyeball, and that the focussing of the eye for near and distant objects was accomplished by the lengthening and shortening of the globe as a whole. The papers describing his experiments were printed in various medical journals at the time, and have been summarized in the opening chapters of his book, *Perfect Sight Without Glasses*.

Whether Dr. Bates was right or wrong in his rejection of the Helmholtz theory of accommodation, I am entirely unqualified to say. My own guess, after reading the evidence, would be that both the extrinsic muscles and the lens play their part in accommodation.

This guess may be correct; or it may be incorrect. I do not greatly care. For my concern is not with the anatomical mechanism of accommodation, but with the art of seeing—and the art of seeing does not stand or fall with any particular physiological hypothesis. Believing that Bates' theory of accommodation was untrue, the orthodox have concluded that his technique of visual education must be unsound. Once again this is an unwarranted conclusion, due to a failure to understand the nature of an art, or psycho-physical skill.

The Nature of an Art

Every psycho-physical skill, including the art of seeing, is governed by its own laws. These laws are established empirically by people who have wished to acquire a certain accomplishment, such as playing the piano, or singing, or walking the tight rope, and who have discovered, as the result of long practice, the best and most economical method of using their psycho-physical organism to this particular end. Such people may have the most fantastic views about physiology; but this will make no difference so long as their theory and practice of psycho-physical functioning remain adequate to their purpose. If psycho-physical skills depended for their development on a correct knowledge of learned physiology, then nobody would ever have learned any art whatsoever. It is probable, for example, that Bach never thought about the physiology of muscular activity; if he ever did, it is quite certain that he thought incorrectly. That, however, did not prevent him from using his muscles to play the organ with incomparable dexterity. Any given art, I repeat, obeys only its own laws; and these laws are the laws of effective psycho-physical functioning, as applied to the particular activities connected with that art.

The art of seeing is like the other fundamental or primary psycho-physical skills, such as talking, walking and using the hands. These fundamental skills are normally acquired in early infancy or childhood by a process of mainly unconscious self-instruction. It takes apparently several years for adequate seeing habits to be formed. Once formed, however, the habit of using the mental and physiological organs of vision correctly becomes automatic—in exactly the same way as does the habit of using the throat, tongue and palate for talking, or the legs for walking. But whereas it takes a very serious mental or physical shock to break down the automatic habit of talking or walking correctly, the habit of using the seeing organs as they should be used can be lost as the result of relatively trivial disturbances. Habits of correct use are replaced by habits of incorrect use; vision suffers, and in some cases the malfunctioning contributes to the appearance of diseases and chronic organic defects of the eyes. Occasionally nature effects a spontaneous cure, and the old habits of correct seeing are restored almost instantaneously. But the majority must consciously reacquire the art which as infants they were able to learn unconsciously. The technique of this process of re-education has been worked out by Dr. Bates and his followers.

Basic Principle Underlying the Practice of Every Art

How can we be sure, it may be asked, that this is the correct technique? The proof of the pudding is in the eating, and the first and most convincing test of the system is that it works. Moreover, the nature of the training is such that we should expect it to work. For the Bates Method is based upon precisely the same principles as those which underlie every successful system ever devised for the teaching of psycho-physical skill. Whatever the art you may wish to learn—whether it be acrobatics or violin playing, mental prayer or golf, acting, singing, dancing or what you will—there is one thing that every good teacher will always say: Learn to combine relaxation with activity; learn to do what you have to do without strain; work hard, but never under tension.

To speak of combining activity with relaxation may seem paradoxical; but in fact it is not. For relaxation is of two kinds, passive and dynamic. Passive relaxation is achieved in a state of complete repose, by a process of consciously "letting go." As an antidote to fatigue, as a method of temporarily relieving excessive muscular tensions, together with the psychological tensions that always accompany them, passive relaxation is excellent. But it can never, in the nature of things, be enough. We cannot spend our whole lives at rest, and consequently cannot be always passively relaxing. But there is also something to which it is legitimate to give the name of dynamic relaxation. Dynamic relaxation is that state of the body and mind which is associated with normal and natural functioning. In the case of what I have called the fundamental or primary psycho-physical skills, normal and natural functioning of the organs involved may sometimes be lost. But having been lost, it may subsequently be consciously reacquired by anyone who has learned the suitable techniques. When it has been reacquired, the strain associated with impaired functioning disappears and the organs involved do their work in a condition of dynamic relaxation.

Malfunctioning and strain tend to appear whenever the conscious "I" interferes with instinctively acquired habits of proper use, either by trying too hard to do well, or by feeling unduly anxious about possible mistakes. In the building up of any psycho-physical skill the conscious "I" must give orders, but not too many orders—must supervise the forming of habits of proper functioning, but without fuss and in a modest, self-denying way. The great truth discovered on the spiritual level by the masters of prayer, that "the more there is of the 'I,' the less there is of God," has been discovered again and again on the physiological level by the masters of the various arts and skills. The more there is of the "I," the less there is of Nature—of the right and normal functioning of the organism. The part played by the conscious "I" in lowering resistance and preparing the body for disease has long been recognized by medical science. When it frets too much, or is frightened, or worries and grieves too long and too intensely, the conscious "I" may reduce its body to such a state that the poor thing will develop, for example, gastric ulcers, tuberculosis, coronary disease and a whole host of functional disorders of every kind and degree of seriousness. Even decay of the teeth has been shown, in the case of children, to be frequently correlated with emotional tensions experienced by the conscious "I." That a function so intimately related to our psychological life as vision should remain unaffected by tensions having their origin in the conscious "I" is inconceivable. And, indeed, it is a matter of common experience that the power of seeing is greatly lowered by distressing emotional states. As one practices the techniques of visual education, one discovers the extent to which this same conscious "I" can interfere with the processes of seeing even at times when no distressing emotions are present. And it interferes, we discover, in exactly the same way as it interferes with the process of playing tennis, for example, or singing—by being too anxious to achieve the desired end. But in seeing, as in all other psycho-physical skills, the anxious effort to do well defeats its own object; for this anxiety produces psychological and physiological strains, and strain is incompatible with the proper means for achieving our end, namely normal and natural functioning.

Chapter 3

Sensing
+ Selecting
+ Perceiving
= Seeing

Before undertaking a detailed description of the techniques employed by Dr. Bates and his followers, I propose to devote a few pages to a discussion of the process of seeing. Such a discussion will serve, I hope, to throw some light on the underlying reasons for these techniques, some of which might otherwise appear inexplicable and arbitrary.

When we see, our minds become acquainted with events in the outside world through the instrumentality of the eyes and the nervous system. In the process of seeing, mind, eyes and nervous system are intimately associated to form a single whole. Anything which affects one element in this whole exercises an influence upon the other elements. In practice, we find that it is possible to act directly only upon the eyes and the mind. The nervous system which connects them cannot be influenced except indirectly.

The structure and mechanism of the eye have been studied in minute detail, and good descriptions of these things can be found in any text book of ophthalmology or physiological optics. I will not attempt to summarize them in this place; for my concern is not with anatomical structures and physiological mechanisms, but with the process of seeing—the process whereby these structures and mechanisms are used to provide our mind with visual knowledge of the external world.

In the paragraphs that follow I shall make use of the vocabulary employed by Dr. C.D. Broad in *The Mind and Its Place in Nature,* a book which for subtlety and exhaustiveness of analysis and limpid clarity of exposition takes rank among the masterpieces of modern philosophical literature.

The process of seeing may be analyzed into three subsidiary processes—a process of sensing, a process of selecting and a process of perceiving.

That which is sensed is a set of *sensa* within a field. (A visual *sensum* is one of the colored patches which form, so to say, the raw material of seeing, and the visual field is the totality of such colored patches which may be sensed at any given moment.)

Sensing is followed by selecting, a process in which a part of the visual field is discriminated, singled out from the rest. This process has, as its physiological basis, the fact that the eye records its clearest images at the central point of the retina, the macular region with its minute *fovea centralis,* the point of sharpest vision. There is also, of course, a psychological basis for selection; for on any given occasion there is generally something in the visual field which it is in our interest to discriminate more clearly than any other part of the field.

The final process is that of perceiving. This process entails the recognition of the sensed and selected *sensum* as the appearance of a physical object existing in the external world. It is important to remember that physical objects are not given as primary data. What is given is only a set of *sensa*; and a *sensum*, in Dr. Broad's language, is something "nonreferential." In order words, the *sensum*, as such, is a mere colored patch having no reference to an external physical object. The external physical object makes its appearance only when we have discriminatively selected the *sensum* and used it to perceive with. It is our minds which interpret the *sensum* as the appearance of a physical object out in space.

It is clear from the behavior of infants that we do not enter the world with full-fledged perceptions of objects. The newborn child starts by sensing a mass of vague, indeterminate *sensa*, which it does not even select, much less perceive as physical objects. Little by little it learns to discriminate the *sensa* that have, for its particular purposes, the greatest interest and significance, and with these selected *sensa* it gradually comes through a process of suitable interpretation to perceive external objects. This faculty for interpreting *sensa* in terms of external physical objects is probably inborn; but it requires for its adequate manifestation a store of accumulated experiences and a memory capable of retaining such a store. The interpretation of *sensa* in terms of physical objects becomes rapid and automatic only when the mind can draw on its past experience of similar *sensa* successfully interpreted in a similar way.

In adults the three processes of sensing, selecting and perceiving are for all intents and purposes simultaneous. We are aware only of the total process of seeing objects, and not of the subsidiary processes which culminate in seeing. It is possible, by inhibiting the activity of the interpreting mind, to catch a hint of the raw *sensum*, as it presents itself to the eyes of the newborn child. But such hints are very imperfect at best, and of brief duration. For the adult, a complete recapture of the experience of pure sensation, without perception of physical objects, is possible, in most cases, only in certain abnormal conditions, when the upper levels of the mind have been put out of action by drugs or disease. Such experiences cannot be introspected while they are going on; but they can often be remembered when the mind has recovered its normal condition. By calling up these memories we can provide ourselves with an actual picture of those processes of sensing, selecting and perceiving, which culminate in the end process of seeing physical objects in the external world.

An Illustration

Here, by way of example, is an account of an experience of my own, while "coming out" of an anesthetic administered in the dentist's chair. Returning awareness began with pure visual sensations completely devoid of significance. These, as I can remember them, were not of objects existing "out there" in the familiar, three-dimensional world of everyday experience. They were just colored patches, existing in and for themselves, unrelated not only to the external world, but also to myself—for the knowledge of self was still wholly lacking, and these meaningless and unattached sense impressions were not *mine*; they simply *were*. This kind of awareness lasted for a minute or two; when the effect of the anesthetic wore off a little further, a notable change took place. The colored patches were no longer sensed merely as colored patches, but became associated with certain objects "out there" in the external three-dimensional world— specifically the façades of houses seen through the window facing the chair in which I was reclining. Attention travelled across the visual field selecting successive parts of it and perceiving these selected parts as physical objects. From being vague and meaningless, the *sensa* had developed into manifestations of definite things belonging to a familiar category and situated in a familiar world of solid objects. Thus recognized and classified, these perceptions (I do not call them "my" perceptions, for "I" had not yet made my appearance on the scene) became immediately clearer, while all sorts of details, unnoticed so long as the *sensa* lacked significance, were now perceived and evaluated. That which was now being apprehended was no longer a set of mere colored patches, but a set of aspects of the known, because remembered, world. Known and remembered by whom? For a time there was no indication of an answer. But after a little while, imperceptibly, there emerged myself, the subject of the experience. And with this emergence there came, as I remember, a further clarification of vision. What had been at first raw *sensa* and had then become, by interpretation, the appearances of known varieties of objects, underwent a further transformation and became objects consciously related to a self, an organized pattern of memories, habits and desires. By becoming related to the self, the perceived objects became more visible, inasmuch as the self, to which they had now entered into relation, was interested in more aspects of external reality than had been the merely physiological being which had sensed the colored patches, and the more developed, but still unself-conscious being which had perceived these *sensa* as appearances of familiar objects "out there" in a familiar kind of world. "I" had now returned; and since "I" happened to take an interest in architectural details and their history, the things seen through the window were immediately thought of as a member of a new category—not merely as houses, but as houses of a particular style and date, and as such possessed of distinguishing characteristics which, when looked for, could be seen even by eyes as inadequate as my own then were. These distinguishing characteristics were now perceived, not because my eyes had suddenly improved, but simply because my mind was once more in a condition to look for them and register their significance.

I have dwelled at some length on this experience, not because it is in any way remarkable or strange, but simply because it illustrates certain facts which every student of the art of seeing must constantly bear in mind. These facts may be formulated as follows:

Sensing is not the same as perceiving.

The eyes and nervous system do the sensing, the mind does the perceiving.

The faculty of perceiving is related to the individual's accumulated experiences, in other words, to memory.

Clear seeing is the product of accurate sensing and correct perceiving.

Any improvement in the power of perceiving tends to be accompanied by an improvement in the power of sensing and of that product of sensing and perceiving which is seeing.

Perception
Determined by Memory

The fact that heightened powers of perception tend to improve the individual's capacity for sensing and seeing is demonstrated, not merely under such abnormal circumstances as I have described, but in the most ordinary activities of everyday life. The experienced microscopist will see certain details on a slide; the novice will fail to see them. Walking through a wood, a city dweller will be blind to a multitude of things which the trained naturalist will see without difficulty. At sea the sailor will detect distant objects which, for the landsman, are simply not there at all. And so on, indefinitely. In all such cases improved sensing and seeing are the result of heightened powers of perceiving, themselves due to the memory of similar situations in the past. In the orthodox treatment of defective vision attention is paid to only one element in the total process of seeing, namely the physiological mechanism of the sensing apparatus. Perception and the capacity to remember, upon which perception depends, are completely ignored. Why and with what theoretical justification, goodness only knows. For in view of the enormous part which mind is known to play in the total process of seeing, it seems obvious that any adequate and genuinely aetiological treatment of defective vision must take account, not only of sensing but also of the process of perceiving, as well as that other process of remembering, without which perceiving is impossible. It is a highly significant fact that, in Dr. Bates' method for re-educating sufferers from defective vision, these mental elements in the total process of seeing are not neglected. On the contrary, many of his most valuable techniques are directed specifically to the improvement of perception and of that necessary condition of perception, memory.

Chapter 4

*Variability of Bodily and
Mental Functioning*

The most characteristic fact about the functioning of the total organism, or of any part of the organism, is that it is not constant, but highly variable. Sometimes we feel well, sometimes we feel poorly; sometimes our digestion is good, sometimes it is bad; sometimes we can face the most trying situations with calm and poise, sometimes the most trifling mishap will leave us irritable and nervous. This non-uniformity of functioning is the penalty we pay for being living and self-conscious organisms, unremittingly involved in the process of adapting ourselves to changing conditions.

The functioning of the organs of vision—the sensing eye, the transmitting nervous system and the mind that selects and perceives—is no less variable than the functioning of the organism as a whole, or of any other part of the organism. People with unimpaired eyes and good habits of using them possess, so to speak, a wide margin of visual safety. Even when their seeing organs are functioning badly, they still see well enough for most practical purposes. Consequently they are not so acutely conscious of variations in visual functioning as are those with bad seeing habits and impaired eyes. These last have little or no margin of safety; consequently any diminution in seeing power produces noticeable and often distressing results.

Eyes can be impaired by a number of diseases. Some of these affect only the eye; in others the impairment of the eye is a symptom of disease in some other part of the body—in the kidneys, for example, or the pancreas, or the tonsils. Many other diseases and many conditions of mild, chronic disorder cause no organic impairment of the eye, but interfere with proper functioning—often, it would seem, by a general lowering of physical and mental vitality.

Faulty diet and improper posture* may also affect vision.

Other causes of poor visual functioning are strictly psychological. Grief, anxiety, irritation, fear, and indeed any of the negative emotions may cause a temporary, or, if chronic, an enduring condition of malfunctioning.

In the light of these facts, which are matters of everyday experience, we are able to recognize the essential absurdity of the average person's behavior, when there is a falling off in the quality of his seeing. Ignoring completely the general condition of his body and his mind, he hurries off to the nearest spectacle shop and there gets himself fitted for a pair of glasses. The fitting is generally done by someone who has never seen him before and who therefore can have no knowledge of him either as a physical organism or as a human individual. Regardless of the possibility that the failure to see properly may be due to temporary malfunctioning caused by some bodily or psychological derangement, the customer gets his artificial lenses and, after a short, sometimes a long, period of more or less acute discomfort, while they are being "broken in," generally registers an improvement in vision. This improvement, however, is won at a cost. The chances are that he will never be able to dispense with what Dr. Luckiesh calls those "valuable crutches," but that, on the contrary, the strength of the crutches will have to be increased as his power of seeing progressively diminishes under their influence. This is what happens when things go well. But there is always a minority of cases

*See Appendix 1

in which things go badly, and for these the prognosis is thoroughly depressing.

In children visual functioning is very easily disturbed by emotion shock, worry and strain. But instead of taking steps to get rid of these distressing psychological conditions and to restore proper habits of visual functioning, the parents of a child who reports a difficulty in seeing immediately hurry him off to have his symptoms palliated by artificial lenses. As light-heartedly as they would buy their little boy a pair of socks or their little girl a pinafore, they have the child fitted with glasses, thus committing him or her to a complete lifetime of dependence upon a mechanical device which may neutralize the symptoms of faulty functioning, but only, it would seem by adding to its causes.

Defective Eyes Capable of Having Flashes of Normal Vision

At an early state in the process of visual re-education one makes a very remarkable discovery. It is this: as soon as the defective organs of vision acquire a certain degree of what I have called dynamic relaxation, flashes of almost or completely normal vision are experienced. In some cases these flashes last only a few seconds; in others, for somewhat longer periods.

Occasionally—but this is rare—the old bad habits of improper use disappear at once and permanently, and with the return to normal functioning there is a complete normalization of the vision. In the great majority of cases, however, the flash goes as suddenly as it came. The old habits of improper use have reasserted themselves; and there will not be another flash until the eyes and their mind have been coaxed back towards that condition of dynamic relaxation, in which alone perfect seeing is possible. To long-standing sufferers from defective vision, the first flash often comes with such a shock of happy amazement that they cannot refrain from crying out, or even bursting into tears. As the art of dynamic relaxation is more and more completely acquired, as habits of improper use are replaced by better habits, as visual functioning improves, the flashes of better vision become more frequent and of longer duration, until at last they coalesce into a continuous state of normal seeing. To perpetuate the flash—such is the aim and purpose of the educational techniques developed by Dr. Bates and his followers.

The flash of improved vision is an empirical fact which can be demonstrated by anyone who chooses to fulfil the conditions on which it depends. The fact that during a flash one may see with extreme clarity objects that, at ordinary times, are blurred or quite invisible, shows that temporary alleviation of mental and muscular strain results in improved functioning and the temporary disappearance of refractive error.

Variable Eyes Versus Invariable Spectacles

Under changing conditions the defective eye can vary the degree of deformation imposed upon it by habits of improper use. This capacity for variation, which may be towards normality or away from it, is mechanically diminished or even inhibited altogether by the wearing of artificial lenses. The reason is simple. Every artificial lens is ground to correct a specific error of refraction. This means that an eye cannot see clearly through a lens unless it is exhibiting exactly that error of refraction which the lens was intended to correct. Any attempt on the part of the spectacled eyes to exercise their natural variability is at once checked because it always results in poorer vision. And this is true even in cases where the eye varies in the direction of normality; for the eye without errors of refraction cannot see clearly through a lens designed to correct an error it no longer has.

It will thus be seen that the wearing of spectacles confines the eyes to a state of rigid and unvarying structural immobility. In this respect artificial lenses resemble, not the crutches to which Dr.

Luckiesh has compared them, but splints, iron braces and plaster casts.

In this context it seems worth while to mention certain recent and revolutionary advances in the treatment of infantile paralysis. These new techniques were developed by the Australian nurse, Sister Elizabeth Kenny, and have been successfully used in her own country and in the United States. Under the old method of treatment the paralyzed muscle groups were immobilized by means of splints and plaster casts. Sister Kenny will have nothing to do with these devices. Instead she makes use, from the first onset of the disease, of a variety of techniques aimed at relaxing and re-educating the affected muscles, some of which are in a spastic condition of over-contraction, while others (incapable of moving owing to the spasm in neighboring muscle groups) rapidly "forget" how to perform their proper functions. Physiological treatment, such as the application of heat, is combined with an appeal to the patient's conscious mind through verbal instruction and demonstration. The results are remarkable. Under the new treatment the recovery rate is from seventy-five to one hundred percent, depending on the site of the paralysis.

Between the Kenny method and the method developed by Dr. Bates there are close and significant analogies. Both protest against the artificial immobilization of sick organs. Both insist on the importance of relaxation. Both affirm that defective functioning can be re-educated towards normality by proper mind-body coordination. And, finally, both work.

Chapter 5

Causes of Visual Malfunctioning: Disease and Emotional Disturbances

In the preceding chapter I spoke of the impairment of visual functioning due, first, to diseases having their seat in the eye itself or elsewhere in the body, and, second, to psychological derangements connected with the negative emotions of fear, anger, worry, grief and the like. It goes without saying that in these cases the restoration of perfect functioning is contingent upon the removal of its physiological and psychological causes of dysfunction. Meanwhile, however, very considerable improvement can almost always be made by the acquisition and practice of the art of seeing.

It can be laid down as a general physiological principle that improvements in the functioning of a part of the body always tend to be followed by organic improvements within that part. In the case of diseases which have their seat in the eye itself, old habits of improper functioning are very often a causative or predisposing factor. Consequently, the acquisition of new and better habits often leads to rapid improvement in the organic condition of the impaired eye.

Even in those cases where the impairment of the eye is only a symptom of a disease having its seat in some other part of the body, the acquisition of habits of proper use will generally produce a certain improvement in the organic condition of the eye.

It is the same with psychological disorders. Perfect functioning can scarcely be expected so long as there is a persistence of the condition of negative emotion which produced the dysfunction. Nevertheless, consistent practice of the art of seeing can do much to improve functioning, even while the undesirable psychological condition persists; and without practice of the art of seeing it will be very difficult, even when the disturbing conditions have passed, to get rid of the habits of improper use contracted while these conditions were present. Moreover, improvement of visual function may react favorably upon the disturbing condition of mind. Most kinds of improper functioning result in nervous tensions. (In the case of farsighted persons, especially those having a tendency to outward squint, the nervous tension is often extreme, and the victim may be reduced to a condition of almost insane restlessness and agitation.) Such nervous tensions aggravate the disturbing psychological conditions. The intensification of the disturbance increases the dysfunction and so heightens the tensions; the heightened tensions further aggravate the disturbing conditions. And so on, in a vicious circle. But luckily there are also virtuous circles. Improvement of functioning relieves the tensions associated with dysfunction, and this relief of tension acts favorably upon the general conditions. Relief of tension will not, of course, get rid of the disturbing conditions; but it may help to make them progressively more bearable and less harmful in their effects on visual function.

The moral of all this is clear. Where there is reason to believe that improper visual functioning is caused, wholly or in part, by disease or disturbing emotional conditions, take all necessary steps to get rid of these causes; but in the meanwhile learn the art of seeing.

Causes of Visual Malfunctioning: Boredom

Another common impediment to good seeing is boredom, which lowers the general bodily and mental vitality, including that of the organs of vision. From a paper by Joseph E. Barmack, entitled

"Boredom and Other Factors in the Physiology of Mental Effort" and published (New York, 1937) in the *Archives of Psychology,* I select a couple of passages which have a certain relevance to our present subject.

"Reports of boredom are accompanied very frequently by reports of increased appreciation of such distracting stimuli as pains, aches, eyestrain, hunger."

The increased appreciation of eyestrain leads to an increased effort to see; and this increased effort, coupled with the increased effort to fix the attention in spite of being bored, results (in a manner which will be explained in the next section) in a lowering of vision and consequent enhanced sense of eyestrain.

In regard to the effect of mental states upon the condition of the body, Mr. Barmack writes as follows. "Where there is boredom, the situation seems unpleasant, because one is responding to it with inadequate physiological adjustments, caused in turn by inadequate motivation."

The converse of this statement is also true. Inadequate physiological adjustments, due to organic or functional defects (in this instance of the organs of seeing) react unfavorably upon motivation by diminishing the individual's desire to perform a given task, because it is so difficult for him to do it well. This in turn enhances the inadequacy of physiological adaptation, and so on in a vicious circle, boredom increasing functional defect and functional defect increasing boredom. The process is clearly illustrated in children suffering from defective vision. Because the hyperope finds reading uncomfortable, he tends to be bored with close work, and his boredom increases the malfunctioning which makes him farsighted. Similarly, the myope is handicapped when playing games or associating with people, whose faces he cannot clearly see at more than a short distance; consequently he is bored with sports and social life, and the boredom reacts unfavorably on his visual defect. An improvement in vision changes the quality of motivation, and reduces the field in which boredom is experienced. Diminished boredom and improved motivation result in improved physiological adjustments and so help forward the improvement of vision.

Once more, the moral is plain. Avoid, if possible, being bored yourself or boring others. But if you can't help being bored or boring, learn the art the seeing for your own benefit, and teach it to your victims for theirs.

Causes of Visual
Malfunctioning:
Misdirected Attention

All the above-mentioned physical and psychological factors making for improper visual functioning are factors that lie, so to speak, outside the process of seeing. We have now to consider an even more fertile source of dysfunction lying within the seeing-process, namely improperly directed attention.

Attention is the indispensable condition of the two mental elements in the total process of seeing; for without attention there can be no selection from the general sense-field and no perception of the selected *sensa* as the appearances of physical objects.

As with all other psycho-physical activities, there is a right way of directing attention, and there is also a wrong way. When attention is directed in the right way, visual functioning is good; when it is directed in the wrong way, proper functioning is interfered with, and the ability to see falls off.

Much has been written on the subject of attention, and many experiments have been performed with a view to measuring its intensity, its span, its effective duration, its bodily correlations. Only a few of these general considerations and particular facts are relevant to our present subject, and I shall therefore confine myself solely to these.

Attention is essentially a process of discrimination—an act of separating and isolating one particular thing or thought from all the other things in the sense field and thoughts in the mind. In the total process of seeing, attention is closely associated with selection; indeed, it is almost identical with that activity.

The various kinds and degrees of attention may be classified in a number of different ways. So far as seeing is concerned, the most significant classification is that which divides all acts of attention into the two main classes of spontaneous attention and voluntary attention.

Spontaneous attention is the kind of attention we share with the higher animals—the unforced act of selective awareness which is determined by the biological necessities of keeping alive and reproducing the species, or by the exigencies of our second nature, in other words, of our habits and established patterns of thought, feeling and behavior. This kind of attention involves no effort when it is shifting and transitory and not much effort when it is prolonged—for spontaneous attention may be prolonged, even in the animals. (The cat lying in wait beside a mouse hole is an obvious example.)

Voluntary attention is, so to speak, the cultivated variety of the wild, spontaneous growth. It is found only in man, and in animals subjected by human beings to some form of training. It is the attention associated with intrinsically difficult tasks, or with tasks which we have to perform even though we don't particularly want to. A small boy studying algebra exhibits voluntary attention—that is, if he exhibits any attention at all. The same boy playing a game exhibits spontaneous attention. Voluntary attention is always associated with effort, and tends more or less rapidly to produce fatigue.

We must now consider the bodily correlations of attention, in so far as these affect the art of seeing. The first and most significant fact is that sensing, selecting and perceiving cannot take place without some degree of bodily movement.

"Without motor elements," writes Ribot, in his classical study, *The Psychology of Attention,* "perception (and it is clear from the context that he includes under this term sensing and selecting as well as perceiving) is impossible. If the eye be kept fixed upon a given object without moving, perception after a while grows dim, and then disappears. Rest the tips of the fingers upon a table without pressing, and the contact at the end of a few minutes will no longer be felt. But a motion of the eye or of the finger, be it ever so slight, will re-arouse perception. Consciousness is only possible through change; change is only possible through movement. It would be easy to expatiate at great length upon this subject; for although the facts are very manifest and of common experience, psychology has nevertheless so neglected the role sustained by movements, that it actually forgot at last that they are the fundamental condition of cognition in that they are the instrument of the fundamental law of consciousness, which is relativity, change. Enough has now been said to warrant the unconditional statement that, where there is no movement, there is no perception."

It is more than fifty years since Ribot enunciated this important truth about the connection between movement and perception. In theory everyone now agrees that Ribot was right; and yet orthodox ophthalmologists have made no effort to discover how this principle could be applied in practice, so as to improve visual functioning. That task was left to Dr. Bates, in whose system the fundamental importance of movement as an aid to seeing is continually stressed.

Meanwhile the researches of the experimental psychologists have confirmed Ribot's categorical conclusion, and furnished theoretical justification for many of the practices and techniques taught by Dr. Bates and his followers.

In the paper already cited, Dr. J.E. Barmack lays it down that "freely shifting attention is an important prop of vital activity. If attention is restricted to an inadequately motivating task, vital activity is apt to be depressed." And the importance of mobility is similarly stressed by Professor Abraham Wolf, in his article on "Attention" in the Encyclopaedia Britannica. "The concentration of attention upon some object of thought may continue for a considerable time among normal people. But what is commonly called an object or a thought is something very complex, having many parts or aspects and our attention really passes from part to part, backwards and forwards all the time. Our attention to what may be seriously called a single thing, affording no opportunities for the movement of attention from part to part, say a small patch of color, cannot be held for more than about a second, without serious risk of falling into a hypnotic trance, or some similar pathological condition." Where seeing is concerned, this continuous movement of attention from part to part of the object under inspection is normally accompanied by a corresponding movement of the physical sensing-apparatus. The reason for this is simple. The clearest images are recorded in the macular area in the center of the retina, and particularly at the minute *fovea centralis*. The mind, as it selects part after part of the object for perception, causes its eyes to move in such a way that each successive part of the object is seen in turn by that portion of the eye which records the clearest image. (Ears have nothing corresponding to the *fovea centralis*; consequently the indispensable shifting of attention within the auditory field does not involve any parallel shifting of the bodily organ. The discriminating and selecting of auditory *sensa* can be done by the mind alone, and do not require corresponding movements of the ears.)

We have seen that, to be effective, attention must be continuously on the move, and that, because of the existence of the *fovea centralis*, the eyes must shift as continuously as the attention of the mind controlling them. But while attention is always associated in normal subjects with continuous eye movements, it is also associated with the inhibition of movements in other parts of the body. Every bodily movement is accompanied by a more or less vague sensation; and when we are trying to pay attention to something, these sensations act as distracting stimuli. To get rid of such distractions we do what we can to prevent our bodies from moving. If the act of attention is accompanied by manual or other activities connected with the object being attended to, we strive to eliminate all movements except those strictly necessary to our task. If we have no task to perform, we try to inhibit all our movements and to keep our bodies perfectly still. We are all familiar with the behavior of an audience at the concert. While the music is being played the people sit without stirring. As the last chord dies away, there breaks out, along with the applause (or apart from it, if the intermission is between two movements of a symphony) a positive tornado of coughs, sneezes and random fidgetings. The explosive intensity of this outburst is an indication of the strength and completeness of the inhibitions imposed by attention to the music. Francis Galton once took the trouble to count the number of bodily movements observable in an audience of fifty persons who were listening to a rather boring lecture. The average rate was forty-five movements a minute, or one fidget, more or less, for each member of the audience. On the rare occasions when the lecturer deviated into liveliness, the fidget-rate declined by upwards of fifty percent.

Inhibition of unconscious activities goes hand in hand with that of conscious movements. Here are some of the findings in regard to respiration and heart beat, as summarized by R. Philip in a paper on *The Measurement of Attention* published (1928) by the Catholic University of America.

"In visual attention respiration is decreased in amplitude, but the rate is sometimes quickened, sometimes slowed; in auditory attention, the rate is always slowed, but the effect upon amplitude is variable. Restricted breathing often gives a slower heart rate, particularly in the first moments of attention. This slowed rate is to be explained from inhibited breathing, rather than from direct influence of attention."

Continuous movement of the eyes, inhibition of movement in the rest of the body—such is the rule where visual attention is concerned. And so long as this rule is observed, and there is no disease or psychological disturbance, visual functioning will remain normal. Abnormality sets in when the inhibition of movement, which is right and proper in the other parts of the body, is carried over to the eyes, where it is entirely out of place. This inhibition of the movement of the eyes—a movement of which we are mainly unconscious—is brought about by a too greedy desire to see. In our over-eagerness we unconsciously immobilize the eyes, in the same way we have immobilized the other parts of the body. The result is that we begin to stare at that part of the sense-field which we are trying to perceive. But a stare always defeats its own object; for, instead of seeing more, a person who has immobilized his sensing apparatus (an act which also immobilizes the closely correlated attention) thereby automatically lowers his power of seeing, which depends, as we have learned, upon the uninterrupted mobility of the sensing eyes and of the attending, selecting and perceiving mind associated with the eyes.

Moreover, the act of staring (since it represents an effort to repress movements which are normal and habitual) is always accompanied by excessive and continuous tension, and this, in its turn, produces a sense of psychological strain. But where there is excessive and continuous tension, normal functioning becomes impossible, circulation is reduced, the tissues lose their resistance and their powers of recovery. To overcome the effects of impaired functioning, the victim of bad seeing habits stares yet harder, and consequently sees less with greater strain. And so on, in a descending spiral.

There is good reason to suppose that improperly directed attention, resulting in the immobilization of the eyes and mind, is the greatest single cause of visual malfunctioning. The reader will notice, when I come to describe them in detail, that many of the techniques developed by Dr. Bates and his followers are specifically aimed at restoring to the eye and mind that mobility without which, as the experimental psychologists all agree, there cannot be normal sensation or perception.

Chapter 6

Relaxation

In this second section I shall describe in some detail a number of beneficial techniques developed by Dr. Bates and other exponents of the art of seeing. Printed instructions can never replace the personal ministrations of a competent teacher; nor is is possible, in a short book, to indicate exactly how much stress should be laid on any given technique in any given case of visual malfunctioning. Every individual has his or her own particular problems. Equipped with adequate knowledge any individual can discover the solution to those problems. But (especially in difficult cases) a gifted and experienced teacher will certainly make the discovery much more expeditiously, and be able to apply his knowledge much more effectively than the sufferer can do for himself. And yet, in spite of all this, printed instructions still have their use. For the art of seeing includes a number of techniques which are profitable to all, whatever the nature and degree of their malfunctioning. Most of these techniques are extremely simple; consequently there is very little danger of their being misunderstood by those who read descriptions of them. A textbook can never be as good as a competent teacher; but it can certainly be better than nothing.

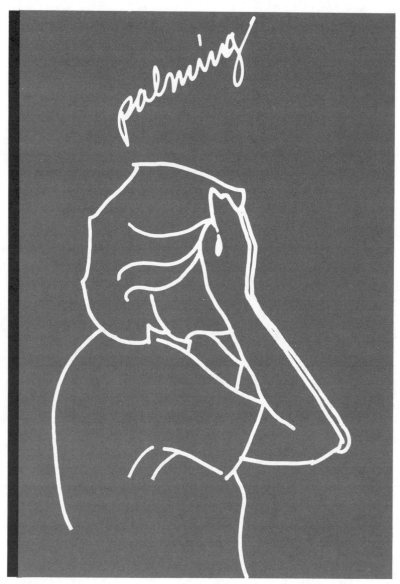

The lower part of the palms should rest upon the cheek bones, the fingers upon the forehead.

Passive Relaxation: Palming

Relaxation, as we have seen, is of two kinds, passive and dynamic. The art of seeing includes techniques for producing either kind—passive relaxation of the visual organs during periods of rest, and dynamic relaxation, through normal and natural functioning in times of activity. Where the organs of vision are concerned, complete passive relaxation can be achieved, but is less beneficial than a mixed state, combining elements of both kinds of relaxation.

The most important of these techniques of (predominantly) passive relaxation is the process which Dr. Bates called "palming." In palming the eyes are closed and covered with the palms of the hands. To avoid exerting any pressure upon the eyeballs (which should never be pressed, rubbed, massaged or otherwise handled) the lower part of the palms should rest upon the cheek bones, the fingers upon the forehead. In this way light can be completely excluded from the eyes, even though the eyeballs remain untouched.

Palming can be done most satisfactorily when one is seated with the elbows resting upon a table, or upon a large, solidly stuffed cushion laid across the knees.

When the eyes are closed and all light has been excluded by the hands, people with relaxed organs of vision find their sense-field uniformly filled with blackness. This is not the case with those whose visual functioning is abnormal. Instead of blackness, these people may see moving grey clouds, darkness streaked with light, patches of color, all in an endless variety of permutations and combinations. With the achievement of passive relaxation of the eyes and the mind associated with them, these illusions of movement, light and color tend to disappear, and are replaced by uniform blackness.

In his book *Perfect Sight Without Glasses*, Dr. Bates advises the candidate for relaxation to "imagine black," while palming. The purpose of this is to come, through imagination, to an actual seeing of black. The technique he describes works satisfactorily in some cases; but in others (and they probably constitute a majority of all sufferers from defective vision) the attempt to imagine black frequently leads to conscious effort and strain. Thus the technique defeats its own object, which is relaxation. Towards the end of his life, Dr. Bates modified his procedure in this matter, and the most successful of his followers have done the same. The person who palms his eyes is no longer told to imagine blackness, but to occupy his mind by remembering pleasant scenes and incidents out of his own personal history. After a period more or less long, according to the intensity of the strain involved, the field of vision will be found to be uniformly black. Thus, the same goal is reached as is done by imagining black—but without risk of making efforts or creating tensions. Care should be taken, when remembering past episodes, to avoid anything in the nature of a "mental stare." By fixing the mind too rigidly upon a single memory image, one may easily produce a corresponding fixation and immobilization of the eyes. (There is nothing surprising or mysterious in this; indeed, in view of the unitary nature of the human organism, or mind-body, this is just the sort of phenomenon one would expect to happen.) To avoid mental staring, with its concomitant fixation of the eyes, one should always while palming remember objects that are in movement.

For example, one may wish to revisit in imagination the scenes of one's childhood. If this is done, one should imagine oneself walking about through the remembered landscape, noticing how its constituent parts change their aspects as one moves. At the same time, the scenes thus evoked may be peopled with human beings, dogs, traffic, all going about their business, while a brisk wind stirs the leaves of the trees and hurries the clouds across the sky. In such a world of phantasy, where nothing is fixed or rigid, there will be no danger of immobilizing the inward eye in a fixed stare; and where the inward eye moves without restraint, the outward, physical eye will enjoy a similar freedom. By using the memory and imagination in the way I have described it is possible to combine, in the single act of palming, the beneficial features of both passive and dynamic relaxation—rest and natural functioning.

This, I believe, is one of the principal reasons why palming is better for the organs of vision than any form of wholly passive relaxation. When the activities of the memory and imagination are completely inhibited, such wholly passive relaxation can be carried, after some practice, to the point where the eyelids and the eyeball itself lose their tone and go soft. This condition is so remote from the normal state of the eyes that its attainment does little or nothing to help in improving vision. Palming, on the contrary, keeps the mental powers of attention and perception at work in the effortless, freely shifting way which is natural to them, at the same time as it rests the eyes.

The other main reasons for the efficacy of palming are of a physical nature. There is refreshment in the temporary exclusion of light, and comfort in the warmth of the hands. Moreover, all parts of the body carry their own characteristic potentials; and it is possible that the placing of the hands over the eyes does something to the electrical condition of the fatigued organs—something that re-invigorates the tissues and indirectly soothes the mind.

Be this as it may, the results of palming are remarkable. Fatigue is rapidly relieved; and when the eyes are uncovered, vision is often noticeably improved, at any rate for a time.

When there is strain and when vision is defective, there can never be too much palming. Many who have experienced its benefits deliberately set aside regular periods for palming. Others prefer to take such opportunities as each day may casually offer, or as their own fatigue may make it urgently necessary for them to create. In even the busiest lives there are blank and unoccupied intervals, which may profitably be used to relax the eyes and mind, and so to gain improved vision for further work. In all cases, the important thing to remember is that prevention is better than cure, and that, by devoting a few minutes to relaxation, one may spare oneself many hours of fatigue and lowered visual efficiency. In the words of Mr. F.M. Alexander, we all tend to be greedy "end-gainers," paying no attention to our "means-whereby." And yet is must be obvious to anyone who will give the subject a moment's thought, that the nature of the means employed will always determine the nature of the end attained. In the case of the eyes and the mind controlling them, means that involve unrelieved strain result in lowered vision and general physical and mental fatigue. By allowing ourselves intervals of the right sort of relaxation, we can improve the means-whereby and so arrive more easily at our end, which is, approximately, good vision and, ultimately, the accomplishment of tasks for which good vision is necessary.

"Seek ye first the kingdom of God and His righteousness, and all the rest shall be added." This saying is as profoundly true on the plane of the psycho-physiological skills as it is upon the planes of spirituality, ethics and politics. By seeking first relaxed visual functioning of the kind that Nature intended us to have, we shall find that all the rest will be added to us, in the form of better sight and heightened powers of work. If, on the contrary, we persist in behaving as greedy and thoughtless end-gainers, aiming directly at better vision (through mechanical devices for neutralizing symptoms) and increased efficiency (through unremitting strain and effort), we shall end by seeing worse and getting less work done.

Where circumstances make it difficult or embarrassing to assume the attitude of palming, it is possible to obtain a certain measure of relaxation by palming mentally—that is, by closing the eyes, imagining that they are covered with the hands and remembering some pleasant scene or episode, as suggested in an earlier paragraph. This should be accompanied by a conscious "letting go" of the eyes—a "thinking of looseness" in relation to the strained and tired tissues. Purely mental palming is not so beneficial as palming which is both mental and physical; but it is a good second-best.

Chapter 7

Blinking and Breathing

It is hard to say whether the kind of relaxation achieved through the techniques described in the present and subsequent chapters is predominantly passive or predominantly dynamic. Luckily, it is of no practical importance how we answer the question. The significant facts about them are that all of them are designed to relieve strain and tension; that all may and should be practiced as relaxation drills in periods specially set aside for the purpose; and that all may and should be incorporated into the everyday business of seeing, so as to produce and maintain the state of dynamic relaxation associated with normal functioning. I shall begin with a brief account of blinking, and its importance in the art of seeing.

Normal and Abnormal
Blinking Habits

Blinking has two main functions: to lubricate and cleanse the eyes with tears; and to rest them by periodically excluding light. Dryness of the eyes predisposes them to inflammation, and is often associated with blurring of vision. Hence the imperative need for frequent lubrication—that is to say, for frequent blinking. Moreover, dust (as everyone knows who has ever cleaned a window) will stick to even the smoothest surface, and render the most transparent material opaque. The eyelids, as they blink, wash the exposed surfaces of the eyes with tears, and prevent them from becoming dirty. At the same time, when blinking is frequent, as it should be, light is excluded from the eyes during perhaps five percent or more of all the waking hours.

Eyes in a condition of dynamic relaxation blink often and easily. But where there is strain, blinking tends to occur less frequently, and the eyelids work tensely. This would seem to be due to that same misdirection of the attention, which causes the improper immobilization of the sensing apparatus. The inhibition of movement, natural and normal in the other parts of the body, is carried over, not only to the eyes, but to their lids as well. A person who stares closes the eyelids only at long intervals. This fact is a matter of such common observation that, when novelists write about a stare, they generally qualify the word with the epithet, "unwinking."

Movement, as the psychologists have long been insisting, is one of the indispensable conditions of sensing and perceiving. But so long as the eyelids are kept tense and relatively immobile, the eyes themselves will remain tense and relatively immobile. Consequently, anyone who wishes to acquire the art of seeing well must cultivate the habit of frequent and effortless blinking. When mobility has been restored to the eyelids, the restoration of mobility to the sensing apparatus will be comparatively easy. Also, the eyes will enjoy better lubrication, more rest, and the improved circulation that is always associated with unstrained muscular movement.

Those who blink too little and too tensely—and they comprise a majority of the sufferers from defective vision—must consciously acquire, or reacquire, the habit of blinking often and easily. This can be done by pausing every now and then to perform a brief blinking-drill—half a dozen light, butterfly blinks; then a few seconds of relaxed closure of the lids; then more blinks, and another closing. And so on for half a minute or a minute. Repeated at frequent intervals (say, every hour or so) these drills will help to build up the habit of frequent blinking during the rest of the day. A person who has become "blink-conscious" will also be conscious of his own tendencies to immobilize the eyes and lids, and will be able to check the incipient stare by frequent and easy closures of the lids. Frequent blinking is especially important for those engaged in any form of difficult and detailed work, requiring close attention. When busy with such tasks, it is fatally easy to fix the eyes and lids, with resulting strain, fatigue, dryness of the cornea, inflammation and impairment of vision. Frequent and easy blinking will often bring a measure of relief that seems out of all proportion to the simplicity of the means employed.

Besides blinking, one may, with advantage, periodically squeeze the eyes tight shut, reinforcing the action of the lids with that of the other facial muscles. This should be done on all occasions when one is tempted to rub the eyes—a barbarous and brutal method of doing with the knuckles what the beautifully adjusted eyelids can do much more safely and just as effectively. It may also be done occasionally, even when there is no itching or other discomfort in the eyes— merely to increase local circulation and stimulate the secretion of tears.

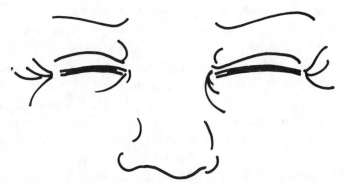

Massage of the eyes themselves is always undesirable; but a gentle rubbing of the temples will often be found soothing and refreshing. Eye fatigue may also be relieved by rubbing and kneading the muscles of the upper part of the nape of the neck. (In certain cases of defective vision, appropriate treatment by a capable osteopath will often produce excellent results.) People who are subject to eye strain may profitably use this rudimentary kind of massage upon themselves, two or three times a day and follow it up by a period of palming.

Normal and Abnormal Breathing Habits

As was pointed out in the first section of this book, experimental psychologists have noted a fairly regular correlation between the state of attentiveness and a modification of the normal rate and amplitude of breathing. To put it more simply, they have noticed that, when we look at something attentively, we tend either to hold our breath for many seconds at a stretch, or alternatively, if we do breathe, to breathe less deeply than at ordinary times. The reason for this is that when we are trying to concentrate our attention, we find that the sounds and the sense of muscular movement, associated with breathing, are sources of distraction. We try to get rid of these distractions, either by breathing less deeply, or by suspending our breathing altogether during relatively prolonged periods of time.

In their strained effort to see, people with defective vision tend to carry this normal interference with breathing to entirely abnormal extremes. Many of them, when paying close attention to something they are particularly anxious to see, behave almost as if they were diving for pearls, and remain for incredibly long periods without drawing breath. But vision depends to a remarkable extent upon good circulation; and circulation can be described as good only when it is sufficient in quantity (which it is not when the mind is under strain and the eyes are in a condition of nervous muscular tension), and at the same time of good quality (which it certainly is not when restricted breathing has left the blood imperfectly oxygenated).

The quantity of circulation in and around the eyes may be increased by means of relaxation, passive and dynamic. The quality can be improved by learning consciously to breathe, even while paying attention. Some of the techniques of relaxation have already been described, and I shall have occasion later on to mention several others. In this subsection our concern is only with breathing.

In correcting abnormal breathing habits, the first thing to do is to become aware that they *are* abnormal. Impress upon yourself the fact that among persons with defective sight there is a regular correlation between attentive looking and a quite unnecessary, indeed positively harmful, interference with breathing. Kept in the back of the mind, this will periodically pop out into consciousness; and if it does this at a time when you are paying close attention to something, the chances are that you will catch yourself behaving as though you were a pearl fisher ten fathoms under the surface of the sea. But you are not a pearl fisher, and the element in which you live is not water, but life-giving air. Therefore, fill your lungs with the stuff—not violently, as though you were doing deep-breathing exercises, but in an easy, effortless way, expiration following inspiration in a natural rhythm. Continue, while breathing in this way, to pay attention to the thing you want to see. (In later chapters of this book I shall describe the proper way of paying attention.) You will find it possible after a little practice to be just as concentratedly attentive when breathing normally, or even rather more deeply than at ordinary times, as it is when behaving like a pearl fisher. In a little while you will find that breathing while paying attention has become habitual and automatic. Any improvement in the quality of circulation is reflected immediately in better vision; and when through relaxation quantity has also been increased, this improvement in vision will be even greater.

In cases of failing sight due to old age or other causes, and in certain pathological conditions of the eye, some doctors, particularly those of the Viennese school, make successful use of mechanical methods for increasing local circulation. Temporary hyperemia of the regions around the eye is produced by dry cupping of the temples, or by the application of leeches, or sometimes by fastening around the neck a specially made elastic collar, so adjusted as to permit the blood to flow freely into the head through the arteries, while reducing the amount to return by slightly constricting the veins. None of these procedures should be tried out except under expert medical advice; nor, indeed, is it necessary in most cases that they should be tried. Relaxation and proper breathing will bring about an equal improvement in circulation, more slowly indeed, but more safely and naturally, and by methods which are entirely under the control of the person employing them. Moreover, the resulting improvement in visual functioning and in the organic condition of the eyes will be the same, whichever means of increasing circulation are employed. The mechanical methods are no better than the self-directed, psychophysical methods here described. Indeed, insofar as they *are* mechanical, they are intrinsically less satisfactory. If I mention them at all, it is merely in order to corroborate the assertion that vision and the organic health of the eyes depend upon adequate circulation.

The extent of this dependence can be demonstrated in a very simple way. As you read, draw a deep breath and then exhale. While the air is being breathed out, you will notice that the print before your eyes becomes perceptibly clearer, blacker and more distinct. This temporary improvement of vision is due to a slight temporary hyperemia in the head; and this, in turn, is due to the slight constriction of the veins in the neck caused by the act of expiration. More than the usual amount of blood is present in and around the eyes— with the result that the sensing apparatus does its work more efficiently, and the mind is given better material with which to do its perceiving and seeing.

Chapter 8

The Eye, Organ of Light

In insects and fishes, in birds and beasts and men, eyes have been developed with the express purpose of responding to light waves. Light is their element; and when they are deprived of light, either wholly or in part, they lose their power and even develop serious diseases, such as the nystagmus of coal miners. This does not mean, of course, that eyes must be perpetually exposed to light. Sleep is necessary to the mind that perceives, and for seven or eight hours at least out of the twenty-four, darkness is necessary to the sensing apparatus. The eyes do their work most easily and efficiently when they are allowed to alternate between good solid darkness and good bright light.

The Current Fear of Light

In recent years there has grown up a most pernicious and entirely unfounded belief that light is bad for the eyes. An organ which for some scores of millions of years has been adapting itself very successfully to sunshine of all degrees of intensity is now

supposed to be incapable of tolerating daylight without the mitiga-
tino intervention of tinted goggles, or lamplight, except when diffused through ground glass or reflected from the ceiling. This extraordinary notion that the organ of light perception is unfitted to stand
light has become popular only in the last twenty years or so. Before
the war of 1914 it was, I remember, the rarest thing to see anyone
wearing dark glasses. As a small boy I would look at a begoggled man
or woman with that mixture of awed sympathy and rather macabre
curiosity which children reserve for those afflicted with any kind of
unusual or disfiguring physical handicap. Today all that is changed.
The wearing of black spectacles has become not merely common, but
creditable. Just how creditable is proved by the fact that the girls in
bathing suits, represented on the covers of fashion magazines in
summer time, invariably wear goggles. Black glasses have ceased to
be the badge of the afflicted, and are now compatible with youth,
smartness and sex appeal.

This fantastic craze for blacking out the eyes had its origin in
certain medical circles, where a panic terror of the ultra-violet radia-
tions in ordinary sunlight developed about a generation back; it has
been fostered and popularized by the manufacturers and vendors of
colored glass and celluloid spectacle frames. Their propaganda has
been effective. In the Western world millions of people now wear
dark glasses, not merely on the beach or when driving their cars, but
even at dusk, or in the dimly lit corridors of public buildings. Need-
less to say, the more they wear them, the weaker their eyes become
and the greater their need for "protection" from the light. One can
acquire an addiction to goggles, just as one can acquire an addiction to
tobacco or alcohol.

This addiction has its origin in the fear of light—a fear which
those who have it feel to be justified by the discomfort they experience when their eyes are exposed to too intense a brightness. The
question arises: why this fear and this discomfort? Animals get on
very happily without goggles; so do primitive men. And even in
civilized societies, even in these days when the virtues of colored
glass are everywhere persuasively advertised, millions of people face

the sunlight without goggles and, so far from suffering any ill effects, see all the better for it. There is every reason to suppose that, physiologically, the eyes are so constructed that they can tolerate illuminations of very high intensity. Why, then, do so many people in the contemporary world experience discomfort when exposed to light even of relatively low intensity?

Reasons for the Fear of Light

There seem to be two main reasons for this state of things. The first is connected with the silly craze for shutting out the light, described in an earlier paragraph. Medical alarmists and the advertisers, who exploit the opinions of these learned gentlemen for their own profit, have convinced large sections of the public that light is harmful to the eyes. This is not true; but the belief that it is true can cause a great deal of harm to those who entertain it. If faith can move mountains, it can also ruin vision—as anyone may see for himself who has watched the behavior of light-fearing people when suddenly exposed to sunshine. They *know* that light is bad for them. Consequently, what grimaces! What frowns! What narrowing of the lids! What screwings-up of the eyes! In a word, what manifest symptoms of strain and tension! Originating in a false belief, the purely mental terror of light expresses itself physically in terms of a strained and thoroughly abnormal condition of the sensing apparatus. Eyes in such a condition are no longer capable of reacting as they should to the external environment. Instead of accepting the sunlight easily and as a blessing, they suffer discomfort and even develop an inflammation of the tissues. Hence more pain and a heightening of fear, a confirmation of the false faith that light is harmful.

There is also another reason for the discomfort which so many people now experience when exposed to light. They may not start with any *a priori* terror of light; but because their seeing organs are strained and defective, owing to habits of wrong use, their eyes and mind may be incapable of reacting normally to external environment. Strong light is painful to the tense, strained seeing organs.

Because it is painful, a fear of light develops in the mind; and this fear becomes, in its turn, a cause of further strain and discomfort.

Casting Out Fear

The fear of light, like all other kinds of fear, can be cast out of the mind; and the physical discomfort experienced when the sensing apparatus is exposed to light can be prevented by means of suitable techniques. When this has been done, it will no longer be necessary to black out the eyes with tinted goggles. Nor is this all. In the process of learning to react to light in a normal and natural way, defective seeing organs can do much to relieve the strain that impairs their visual power. Acquiring normal reactions to light is one of the essential procedures in the art of seeing. Appropriate drill in connection with sunlight will produce a valuable kind of passive relaxation; and the power so acquired of dealing easily and effortlessly with the strongest illuminations can be carried over into active life, to become an element in that dynamic relaxation of the seeing organs, without which there can never be perfect vision.

In all cases where light causes discomfort, the first thing to do is to cultivate an attitude of confidence. We must bear steadily in mind that light is not harmful, at least in any degree of intensity we are ever likely to meet with; and that, if in fact it produces discomfort, the fault is ours for being afraid of it, or for having habitually used our eyes in the wrong way.

Practical Techniques

Confidence in the harmlessness of light should be translated into practice by a process of gradual habituation. If the eyes shrink from sunlight when open, start by accustoming them to sunlight when they are closed. Sitting comfortably, lean back and "letting go and thinking looseness," close the eyes and turn them towards the sun. To avoid internal staring and the possibility of too prolonged an exposure to the light of any given portion of the retina, move the head gently but fairly rapidly from side to side. A lateral swing of a few inches will be quite sufficient, so long as it is kept up continuously.

In some persons sunning of the eyes will produce discomfort even when the lids are closed. Where this is the case, it will be as well to start by directing the eyes at the sky, and not directly at the sun. When the light of the sky seems tolerable, one may turn for short periods to the sun. As soon as any discomfort is felt, one should turn away, palm the eyes for a little, and then start again. The closed lids may be sunned for several minutes at a stretch (with brief interruptions for palming, if the need of it is felt); and the process should be repeated several times in the course of the day.

After a very little while most people will find that they can, without discomfort, take the sunlight upon the open eyes. The most satisfactory procedure is as follows. Cover one eye with the palm of the hand and, taking care to swing the head from side to side as before, allow the other eye to travel back and forth three or four times across the sun, blinking rapidly, lightly and easily as you do so. Then cover the eye that has been exposed to the sunlight and repeat the same process with the other eye. Alternate for a minute or so; then palm until the after-images disappear. When the eyes are uncovered, it will generally be found that vision has distinctly improved, while the organs feel relaxed and suffused with a warm sense of well-being.

When the open eyes are sunned one at a time, in the manner described above, the light seems far less dazzling than when both are sunned simultaneously. Because the illumination seems more intense, simultaneous sunning of both eyes may result in involuntary shrinking, which is then overcome by an effort of will that results, in its turn, in a state of tension. This condition may postpone the achievement of the complete relaxation which should normally follow the process of sunning. Nevertheless, those who wish to sun both eyes simultaneously may do so in moderation without any fear of harm. It may be noted that the process is accompanied, at first, by a copious discharge of tears and followed by after-images brighter and more lasting than those which attend the sunning of each eye separately. The tears are refreshing, and the after-images soon disappear with palming. On the whole, however, the method of sunning one eye at a time is to be preferred.

Harmlessness of Sunning

The enemies of Dr. Bates' method are fond of telling hair-raising stories about the effects of sunning the eyes. Those who do it are solemnly warned that they will go blind, either at once or (when in fact this doesn't happen) at some future date. From personal experience, as well as from fairly extensive enquiries among people who have taught and practiced the technique, I am convinced that these stories are wholly untrue. When the eyes are sunned in the manner described in the preceding paragraphs, no harmful effects ever follow. On the contrary, the organs are agreeably relaxed, circulation is speeded up, and the vision is improved. Moreover, many forms of inflammation, both of the eye and its lids, tend to clear up very rapidly when the eyes are sunned. There is nothing particularly surprising about these facts. Sunlight is a powerful germicide and, used in moderation, it acts as a valuable therapeutic agent when directed on the human body. There is no reason why it should not act upon the eyes in the same beneficial way as it acts on the other external organs.

The sun produces harmful effects upon the eyes only when people stare fixedly at it. For example, after following the phases of an eclipse, many persons report a temporary impairment of vision, mounting sometimes to partial or even complete blindness. In almost all cases, the condition disappears after a short time, leaving the sufferer none the worse. Among the many thousands who have used the technique developed by Dr. Bates and his followers, a very few have had a similar experience. Neglecting their teachers' advice to keep the head continuously swinging from side to side, they have stared fixedly at the sun. If the results are bad, they have only themselves to blame.

The truth of the matter is that like everything else in the world, sunlight is good for us in reasonable quantities, bad when taken to excess or in the wrong way. If people are foolish enough to eat ten pounds of strawberries at a sitting, or swallow a quart of castor oil, or take a hundred aspirin tablets, they will have to suffer for their folly. Nevertheless, strawberries, castor oil and aspirin are freely sold. The fools must take their chance. It is the same with sunlight. Every summer a great many silly people sunbathe to the point of burning their skin, running a high fever, and even enlarging their spleens. Nevertheless, sun bathing is permitted and encouraged because it is pleasant and beneficial for people who do it reasonably. So too with the eyes. In spite of all the good advice that may be given, some imbeciles will stare fixedly at the sun and so temporarily impair their vision. This is no reason for discouraging those who have the sense to sun their eyes wisely from undertaking a practice which will certainly do them good.

Those who have learned to take the sun on the closed and open eyes, will note a progressive diminution of their susceptibility to glare and bright illuminations. The fear of light and the discomfort caused by light will vanish, and along with them will go the tinted goggles, the frowns and grimaces, and the strain that is always associated with fear and discomfort.

To maintain normal reactions to light one should carry over into active life a modified version of the sunning technique, which is practiced during periods especially set aside for the purpose. If the light seems unpleasantly bright when one goes out of doors, one should close the eyes for a moment, "let go and think looseness," then reopen as gently and relaxedly as possible. After this the eyes should be raised to the sun, which may be taken for a few seconds on the closed lids and afterwards (always with a swing of the head), on the open eyes. When one looks down again, the brightness of the world around will seem very tolerable, and there will be no sense of strain or tension. These procedures should be repeated at frequent intervals when one is out of doors on a bright day. They will help to keep the eyes in a state of dynamic relaxation and to improve the vision.

At night one may use a bright source of artificial light in lieu of the sun. For this purpose, as well as for reading, I have found a 150-watt spot- or flood-light very useful. These bulbs, which are like self-contained headlamps, with a curved and silvered back and a circular transparent front, through which the concentrated beam of light is projected, will give a thousand foot-candles at three or four feet. Using the same procedure as with the sun, one may take this light on the closed and open eyes. Improved relaxation, circulation and vision follow exactly as with the sun. Those who wish to increase the illumination may do so by reflecting the light from a spot-lamp into their eyes by means of a convex shaving mirror. At the focus of the mirror there will be warmth and illumination not greatly inferior to that of the sun itself, when looked at on a bright summer's day.

Chapter 9

Central Fixation

In the present chapter and the two which follow I shall give an account of certain procedures designed to encourage mobility in the defective organs of vision. For more than half a century, as we have seen, experimental psychologists have proclaimed that adequate cognition of the external world depends upon movement. This fact is, obviously and on the face of it, enormously significant for vision. And yet, for some inexplicable reason, orthodox ophthalmologists have never paid the smallest attention to it. As a class, they have been, and still are, content to prescribe crutches for the mechanical palliation of symptoms, and to leave the matter at that. The first person to devote any serious thought to this manifestly important problem was Dr. W.H. Bates—and all he got for his pains was the professional cold shoulder and the reputation of being a crank, or even a quack.

Before describing any of the procedures designed to encourage habits of mobility, I shall give a brief account of the mental and physiological conditions which make such procedures necessary. As explained in the first section of this book, attention is naturally mobile, and shifts continually from one part of the apprehended physical object to another part, one aspect of the thought under consideration to another aspect. Where seeing is concerned, this continuous shifting of the mind is normally accompanied by continuous shifting of the sensing apparatus. The reason for this must be sought in the structure of the eye, which records perfectly clear images only at the central portion of the retina known as the *macula lutea*, with its point of sharpest precision, the *fovea centralis*.

This rule, that we see best only that small area at which we are looking directly, out of the center of sight, has one important exception. At night when there is a minimum of light we do our best and clearest sensing with the outer portions of the retina. This fact was discovered centuries ago by the astronomers, who found that when looking directly at the constellation they could see only the brighter stars, whereas, when they looked somewhat to one side of it, they could detect other stars of smaller magnitude. In the words of the eminent French physicist, François Arago, "in order to see a very dimly lighted object, it is necessary not to look at it." For this reason, when trying to find your way in the dark, you should not look straight ahead; for then you will not see the dimmer objects immediately in front of you. If, on the contrary, you turn your head, first to one side, then to the other, you will see what is directly in front of you "out of the corner of your eye."

Exactly the opposite is the case where vision in the daytime, or under bright artificial illumination, is concerned. In these circumstances (and all that follows applies to vision under good illumination), one senses and sees best only that portion of the visible environment which throws its image upon the *macula* and *fovea*: images recorded by the outer portions of the retina are less distinct as to form, and less accurate as to color, than those recorded by the minute central area.

At average reading distance from the eyes—say fourteen inches—one can easily see the whole page of a book. But the area seen with greatest clarity will be a circle of about half an inch in diameter, while the maximum degree of precision will be confined to a single letter at the center of that circle. This single letter represents that part of the total visible environment, whose image falls, at a given moment, upon the *fovea centralis*; the half-inch circle, that part, whose image falls upon the *macula* surrounding the *fovea centralis*. All the rest of the printed page gets recorded by the outer portions of the retina, and is consequently sensed less clearly.

Because of the existence of this central area of clearer sensing, the mobility of attention necessarily entails a corresponding mobility of the eyes. As the mind shifts its attention to a given part of the regarded object, the eyes are moved automatically and unconsciously, so that the part being attended to shall be the part most clearly sensed—or, to put the matter in physiological terms, so that the light rays reflected from the part that is being attended to shall fall directly upon the *macula* and *fovea centralis*. When this happens we are said to be sensing with central fixation. In order to sense every part of an object with central fixation, or in other words, with maximum clarity, the eye must make an enormous number of minute and rapid shifts from point to point. When it fails to shift, it fails to see all parts of the object with central fixation and therefore with maximum clarity.

Mobility, then, is the normal and natural condition of the selecting and perceiving mind; and, because of the need for central fixation, mobility is also the normal and natural condition of the sensing eye. During infancy and childhood most people learn unconsciously to keep their eyes and mind in the condition of mobility, and to do their sensing with central fixation. But unfortunately, for any one of a great variety of reasons, the habits of proper use may be lost. In one way or another, the conscious "I" interferes with natural and normal functioning. The result is that attention comes to be directed fixedly, instead of with a continuous easy movement from point to point, while the eyes cease to shift, and develop a stare. Malfunctioning produces mental and physical strains, which, in their turn, produce more malfunctioning. Owing to strain and malfunctioning the sensing apparatus undergoes distortion, and errors of refraction and other undesirable physical conditions result. Vision deteriorates, and as the bad habits of use become ingrained with time, the eyes (above all, when fitted with spectacles) lose more and more of their power of self-regulation and resistance to disease.

That staring should always be accompanied by strain and an impairment of vision is not in the least surprising. For when people stare, they try to see every part of a large area as clearly as every other part. But the structure of the eye is such that it *cannot* sense every part of the area as clearly as it senses that one small part which is being looked at with central fixation—in other words, that part whose image falls upon the *macula* and *fovea centralis*. And the nature of the mind is such that it *cannot* do a proper job of perceiving, unless its attention is continually shifting from point to point of the regarded object. To stare is to ignore these necessary conditions of normal sensing and normal seeing. In his greedy anxiety to achieve his end, which is to do the greatest possible amount of good seeing in the shortest possible time, the starer neglects the only means whereby this end can be achieved. Instead he tries to do the impossible. The results are just as bad as one would expect them to be—strain, with consequent errors of refraction and poor vision.

Occasionally the habit of central fixation is never acquired, most often owing to diseases of the eye during infancy. In the great majority of cases, however, it is acquired, along with the other habits of normal use, and only lost at a later date—owing, generally, to the interference of the conscious "I," whose fears and worries, whose cravings and griefs and ambitions are forever interfering with the normal functioning of the physical organs, the nervous system and the mind. When the habit of central fixation has been lost for some time, the *macula* and *fovea* seem to lose some of their natural sensibility through disuse. At the same time the habit of trying to sense objects equally clearly with all parts of the retina leads to an overstimulation of some or all of the eccentric areas, which do their best to increase their sensibility in order to respond to this stimulation. Sometimes this process goes so far that a person will, so to speak, manufacture for himself a false *macula* somewhere on the outer edges of his retina. When this happens, he gets his clearest vision, not when looking straight in front of him, but only when the object is regarded at an angle. This sideways vision can never be anything like so clear as normal vision in the central, macular area. But owing to the *macula's* loss of strength of long-established bad habits, it is the best vision that such an eye and mind can have.

In the majority of cases, however, the loss of the good habits of mobility and central fixation, and the acquisition of the bad habit of staring, or trying to see every part of a large area equally well, do not result in this extreme degree of eccentric fixation. The starer still looks straight ahead. But because he tries to see everything equally well, he reduces the sensibility of his *macula* and *fovea* and builds up an undesirable and abnormal relationship between the perceiving mind and the peripheral areas of the retina, which are now used for sensing as much as, or more than, the central areas. Eccentric fixation is diffused over the whole retina instead of being confined, as in the extreme cases, to a false *macula* at one particular point.

Without central fixation and mobility there cannot be normal vision. Hence the great importance of procedures which teach the normal-sighted person how to preserve the good habits, on which (though he generally does not know it) his good sight depends, and which help the person with defective vision to overcome the bad habits responsible for his bad sight. For those who have never learned central fixation, and for those whose eccentric fixation is extreme, the services of a skilled and experienced teacher will probably be indispensable. The rest, if they are shown how, can do much to help themselves. It is for them that I describe the simple, but effective, techniques which follow.

Chapter 10

Methods of Teaching the Eyes and Mind to Move

Central fixation can be taught directly by methods which permit the pupil to experience the fact that he cannot see every part of a large area with equal clarity. Or it may be taught indirectly by methods which build up habits of mobility—methods which compel the mind to shift its attention and the eye to shift its area of greatest sensitivity from point to point of the regarded object.

Use of the direct method entails a certain danger of increasing the strains from which the pupil already suffers. It seems best, therefore, to approach the goal indirectly. Just as, in the case of palming, the best way to see black is not to try to see it, but to remember pleasant scenes and events out of the past, so the best way to achieve central fixation is not to try to see one small area better than all others, but to cultivate the mobility which is the necessary condition for seeing successive small areas of an object with maximum clarity. Accordingly, I shall begin by describing a number of procedures for increasing the mobility of the eyes and mind; and only when this has been done shall I give an account of methods aimed directly at making the pupil conscious of central fixation. Those whose sight is defective will be well advised to follow the same order in their educational practice. First learn to keep the eyes and the attention in constant easy movement; then, when movement has reactivated them, learn consciously to recognize the manifestations of central fixation and, by recognizing them, to increase their intensity.

Swinging

Whenever we move, objects in the external world appear to move in the opposite direction. Those which are nearest to us seem to move most rapidly, and the rate of apparent movement diminishes with the increase of distance from the eyes, so that objects at a great distance seem to be almost stationary, even when viewed from an express train or a speeding car.

The various procedures, to which Dr. Bates gave the name of "swinging," are primarily designed to make the person who practices them aware of this apparent movement of external objects and, by this means, to encourage a condition of free mobility in the sensing apparatus and the controlling mind. Where such mobility exists, psychological and ocular tensions are relaxed, staring is replaced by rapidly shifting central fixation, and there is a marked improvement in vision.

It is possible to invent and practice a great number of swings; but all of them are variations on one or another of a few fundamental types, which alone will be described.

The Short Swing should be performed while standing in front of a window, or in a doorway, or anywhere else where one can arrange to look past some nearby object at some more distant object. For example, the upright bar of a window frame may serve as the nearby object, while a tree or part of a house on the other side of the street will serve as the more distant object. Inside a room the nearby object can be a tall standard lamp, or a piece of string hanging from the ceiling light, while a picture on the wall, or an ornament on the mantelpiece will do for the more distant object. Standing with the feet about eighteen inches apart, one should swing the body, regu-

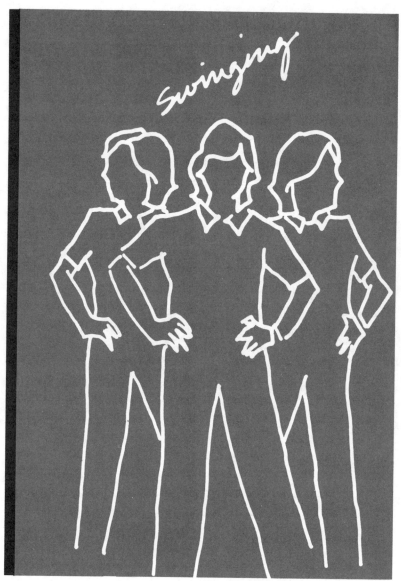

With the feet about eighteen inches apart . . . swing the body . . . from side to side . . . on to each foot alternately.

larly, gently and not too rapidly, from side to side, throwing the weight on to each foot alternately. The swing should not be wide—less than a foot in all is quite sufficient—and the head should not be turned in relation to the shoulders, but should remain looking straight ahead, moving in unison with the trunk. As one swings to the right, the nearby object (say the window bar) will appear to move to the left across the more distant object. As one swings to the left, it will appear to move to the right. This apparent movement should be noted during a number of swings; then the eyes should be closed. Still swinging from side to side, visualize the apparent movement of the window bar across the tree at the end of the garden or the house across the street. Then open again and, during a few more swings, watch the real bar as it moves back and forth. Close again and visualize. And so on for a minute or two, or longer.

This procedure has several advantages. It makes the mind aware of movement and, so to say, friendly to it. It helps to break the defective eye's bad habit of staring. It produces automatically a shifting of attention and of the *fovea centralis*. All these contribute directly to the dynamic relaxation of the organs of seeing. An indirect contribution to the same result comes from the rhythmic movement of swinging, which acts upon mind and body in the same soothing way as do the movements of the cradle and the rocking chair.

To these soothing effects of the Short Swing, the Long Swing adds direct and beneficial action upon the spine by gentle and repeated twisting. When practicing this swing, one stands with the feet apart, as before; but instead of confining the movement of the body to a pendulum-like short sway, one swings in a wider arc, turning the trunk upon the hips and the head upon the shoulders as one does so. As one swings to the left, the weight is thrown on the left foot, while the heel of the right is lifted. Conversely, the left heel is lifted as one turns to the right. The eyes, as they travel from one side to the other, cover an arc of one hundred and eighty degrees, or even more, and the external world seems to oscillate back and forth in a wide sweep. No attempt should be made to pay attention to anything in the eyes' moving sense-field. The attitude of mind, while one is practicing this swing, should be one of complete passivity and indifference. One just "lets the world go by" without caring, without even making any effort to perceive what it is that is going by. The selecting and perceiving mind is out of action, and one is down to pure sensing—a physiological organism taking a holiday from the conscious "I."

Such a holiday from the self is extremely restful. Moreover, since it is generally the conscious "I" that is responsible for poor seeing (either through harboring negative emotions, or through misdirecting its attention, or in some other way ignoring Nature's rules for normal visual functioning) this temporary inhibition of the self's activities is helpful in breaking the old habits of improper use and clearing the ground for the building up of new and better habits. In the Long Swing, the sensing apparatus temporarily escapes from its bondage to a mind that misuses it by immobilizing it into a rigid stare, and learns once more how to function in a condition of free and unstrained mobility.

A variant of the Short Swing, which may be practiced while sitting and in an inconspicuous manner, has been called the Pencil Swing. In this swing, the nearby object is a pencil (or one's own forefinger will do just as well) held vertically about six inches in front of the nose. Swinging the head from side to side, one notes the apparent movement of the pencil across the more distant features of one's environment. The eyes should be closed from time to time, and this apparent movement should be followed with the inward eye of the imagination. When the eyes are opened, they may be focused alternately on the pencil and on the more distant objects across which it seems to pass.

Swinging can and should be carried over from the periods especially set aside for it into the activities of daily life. Perfect vision is impossible without continuous movement of the sensing apparatus and the attention; and it is by cultivating an awareness of the apparent movements of external objects that the staring eyes and immobilized mind can most easily and rapidly be educated out of their sight-impairing habits. Hence, for those with defective vision, the importance of applying the principle of the swing in every variety of visual situation.

To begin with, whenever you move, let the world go by and be aware of its going by. Note, as you walk or travel by car or bus, the approach and passing of trees, houses, lamp-posts, pavements. Indoors, when you turn your head, be conscious of the way in which nearby objects move across more distant objects. By becoming conscious of the seeming mobility of the environment, you increase the mobility of the eyes and mind and so create the conditions for better vision.

Other Aids to Mobility

Swinging is of fundamental importance in the re-establishment of normal visual functioning, and should be practiced as much as possible. But there are also other procedures for cultivating habits of mobility and, indirectly, of central fixation. Here are a few of them.

Throw up a rubber ball with the right hand, and catch it, as it falls, in the left. Or, better, take a ball in either hand, throw up that in the right hand and, while it is in the air, transfer the ball in the left hand to the right hand, then use the left hand to catch the other ball as it comes down. By means of this rudimentary form of juggling one can impart to simple ball throwing a continuous easy rhythm, not present when a single ball is used. The eyes should be on the ball as it is thrown up by the right hand, should follow it up to the top of its trajectory and down again till it is caught by the left hand. (They should *not* stare up into the sky, waiting for the ball to appear within their field of vision.) After a long spell of close work, a brief interlude of this simple juggling will do much to loosen and relax the eyes.

Out of doors, this procedure can be used, not only to remind the eyes to move, but also to establish habits of light tolerance. Start by throwing the ball up against a dark background, such as a tree. Then move so that the ball has to be watched as it traverses the less brightly illuminated portions of the sky. "Think looseness" as you watch it rise and fall, and blink frequently. Then, as the eyes and mind become accustomed to the light, move again, so that the ball has a yet brighter background. The last two or three throws may be made while one is almost facing the sun.

Dice and dominoes may also be used to restore to eyes and mind the mobility without which there can be no proper central fixation, and consequently no normal seeing.

Take three or four dice, throw them on a table, glance quickly from one to another and then, after a second, turn away or close the eyes and name the numbers appearing on their upper faces. If the game is played by two people (as it always must be in the case of children), the instructor should throw the dice, give the pupil a second in which to glance from one to the other, then cover them with his hand and ask for the numbers. This procedure encourages rapid shifting of the attention and the eyes, and at the same time stimulates the interpreting mind in ways which will be described when we come to the subject of "flashing."

Dominoes can also be used to break the habit of staring, and to spur the eyes and mind into the indispensable condition of mobility. Procure a set of dominoes—preferably a set which goes up to double nine, or even to double twelve. Arrange a random selection of the dominoes in, say, three rows of eight or ten each, within the lid of a cardboard box. Wedge them tightly, or glue them into place, so that the lid may be handled without upsetting the dominoes. Stand the lid on edge upon a table, so that the mosaic of dominoes faces you, as you sit at a convenient distance regarding them. Alternatively, if distance vision is beyond your powers, hold the lid in your hand, where the dominoes can be easily seen, increasing the distance as vision improves. Now, as rapidly as you can, name the numbers in the upper halves of the first row of dominoes; then in the lower halves; then in the upper and lower halves, successively, of the other rows. Do this without any thought of test-passing, with mind relaxed and eyes easily moving from domino to domino, and blinking at frequent intervals. Close the eyes for a few seconds between each row. Then start again, and name the number of dots, first, in each horizontal line of every figure on the upper and lower halves of the dominoes, next in each vertical line, next in the diagonals. Then complicate the procedure a little by counting the total number of dots in the vertical lines of the upper and lower figures of each domino taken together.

Valuable in all cases of defective vision associated with strain and staring, these domino drills, together with the others which will be described in the chapter on "flashing," are particularly useful in cases of astigmatism.

Astigmatism occurs when the radius of curvature of the cornea is not the same in all meridians. Light rays passing through this distorted medium are focused in an irregular way. In many sufferers the condition shows a considerable measure of variability. Spectacles tend to fix the cornea rigidly in that particular condition of distortion present at the moment of the oculist's examination. Consequently there is little hope of recovery, so long as one wears artificial lenses. But if the astigmatic person will discard his artificial lenses, learn the art of passive and dynamic relaxation, and cultivate habits of mental and ocular mobility, he can do much to diminish, or even altogether eliminate his disability. Dominoes are very easy to see; consequently the rapid shifting of eyes and mind, encouraged by the domino drills, is almost effortless. Tension is released, and at the same time as the eyes move from dot to dot, an enormous number of acts of sensing are performed in this relaxed condition through every part of the cornea. This seems to have the effect of "ironing out" the distortions of the cornea. Exactly how, we do not know. But if, as seems likely, the disability was originally due to mental and muscular tensions, there is no cause for surprise if the disability should disappear when the sufferer has learned the art of sensing and perceiving without tension. Anyhow, the fact remains that astigmatic persons see distinctly better after the domino drills than before. As old habits of visual functioning are broken down and replaced by new and better habits, the improvements tends to become permanent.

The "ironing-out" process can often be accelerated by a procedure which may be described as a kind of concentrated or streamlined version of the domino drills. Take the lid, in which the rows of dominoes have been firmly fixed, and, holding it in both hands three or four inches before the face, move it backwards and forwards horizontally. This side-to-side movement should not be greater than six or eight inches, and should be accompanied by a corresponding movement of the head in the opposite direction. Thus, when the lid is moved to the left, the head should be turned slightly to the right, and vice versa. No effort should be made to see the numbers on the individual dominoes, and the combined movement of lid and head should be just great enough to create the illusion that one is not looking at separate dots, but at more or less continuous lines, created by the apparent running together of the dots. After a minute or two of this horizontal swinging, the direction of movement should be changed to the vertical plane. Hold the lid with its long axis at right angles to the floor, and move it up and down, accompanying the movement of the hands with a movement of the head in an opposite direction, exactly as in the horizontal swing.

These exercises may seem rather odd, undignified and pointless. But the significant thing about them is that (in conjunction with the other procedures here described) they have helped many astigmatic people to improve their vision, first temporarily and later permanently.

Chapter 11

Flashing

The procedure which Dr. Bates called "flashing" is important for what it does to foster mobility, and to increase the powers of the perceiving and interpreting mind.

Flashing may be described as the antithesis of staring. Instead of fixing the object with one's regard, instead of immobilizing eyes and mind, and straining to see all parts of it equally well at the same time, one glances quickly at it (flashes it), then closes the eyes and remembers what has been sensed in the course of this rapid dart into the unknown.

After a little practice in flashing, one makes the interesting discovery that the sensing apparatus takes in a good deal more than the perceiving mind is aware of—especially when the perceiving mind has built up bad habits of strain and effort. There is a sense in which we see without knowing it. It will be worthwhile, I think, to devote a few paragraphs to the discussion of this "unconscious vision"; for the subject is of considerable theoretical interest, as well as of great practical importance.

Unconscious Vision

"Unconscious vision" is a somewhat inaccurate expression, which is applied to several distinct classes of phenomena.

There is, to begin with, the "unconscious vision" we have when we make a rapid reflex movement to avoid some danger, which the eyes sense and the muscles react to before the mind has had time to interpret the menacing *sensum* as a potentially dangerous external object. In such cases the nervous system works more quickly than the mind, which does not perceive and consciously see until after the danger-avoiding reaction has been initiated. During a fraction of a second there has been unconscious vision and unconscious muscular activity.

Of a similar nature is the kind of "unconscious vision" exhibited by a man who threads his way through traffic or walks across difficult country while engaged in conversation or sunk in thought. He has no distinct conscious awareness of the objects around him, and yet his body behaves as though he were aware—stopping and going, turning and avoiding obstacles, just as it would do, if his mind were on the problem of walking with safety, instead of being on his talk or his thoughts. In this case the mind is in a position at any moment to become fully aware of what is being sensed, and occasionally it actually does become aware. In the intervals, however, there is a measure of unconscious vision—of sensing with a minimum of perceiving.

Finally, there is that most normal and commonplace kind of unconscious vision, which we have, at any given moment, of all those parts of the sense field which we do not select for the purpose of perception. The world is filled with an infinity of objects; but at any given moment our concern is only with a very few of them. From the total visual field we select those *sensa* which happen to interest us, and leave the rest unattended to and unperceived. Where vision is normal, it is always physiologically and psychologically possible for us to select the *sensa* which in fact we do not choose to attend to or perceive. This type of unconscious vision is, in the last analysis, voluntary; if we don't consciously see it is simply because we don't want to see, because it doesn't suit us to see.

There are other cases, however, in which the unconsciousness is involuntary, in which the mind is incapable of making itself aware of what the eyes are sensing. When this happens, we look, but do not see. This may be due to the fact that nothing is sensed, or that the *sensa* are so extremely indistinct that they cannot possibly be interpreted. But this is by no means always the case. Sometimes sensing takes place, and the *sensa* are sufficiently distinct to be used for perceiving with. But in fact they are not so used; and though theoretically we might see what we look at, actually we do not see it. In such cases there is always a measure of ocular and mental strain, which is often related (primarily as cause and secondarily as consequence) to some habitual error of refraction. It is true that the unperceived *sensa* belonging to persons in such a condition of strain are more or less faint and indistinct. Nevertheless they *can* be interpreted and perceived as appearances of external objects. The fact that they are not so interpreted and perceived is due to the condition of strain, which interposes a kind of barrier between the sensing eyes and the perceiving mind.

Now, *sensa* (as Dr. Broad has concluded after considering all the available evidence) always leave "mnemic traces" of the kind that may subsequently be revived and give rise to a memory image. (Concerning the nature of these mnemic traces, or "engrams," nobody as yet knows anything at all. They may be purely physical, or purely psychological, or simultaneously physical and psychological. The only thing we are justified in assuming about them is that they exist and can give rise, under favorable conditions, to memory-images.)

The experience of those who have undertaken a course of visual re-education adds further weight to the evidence for the hypothesis that *sensa* leave traces, and can therefore be remembered, even when, at the time, they were unperceived by the conscious mind. When people with defective vision take a flashing glance at some object, it often happens that they do not see it at all, or see it only as a dim blur.

But on turning away and closing the eyes, they frequently discover that they have a memory-image of what was sensed. Often this image is so extremely tenuous that they are hardly conscious of its being there at all. But if they stop anxiously trying to bring it up into consciousness, and just make a random guess at its nature, it very frequently turns out that the guess is correct. From this we may conclude that it is possible for us to remember what we sensed, but did not see, provided always that the mental tensions associated with the conscious "I" are relaxed, either through hypnosis, or by other, less drastic methods.

This final proviso is of the highest practical significance. Strain, as I have said, erects a barrier between the sensing eyes and the perceiving mind. But if the strained organs of vision are relaxed, as they can be by palming, sunning and swinging, the barrier is lowered; and though it may not be possible at first to perceive what the sensing apparatus takes in, as it regards a given external object, it becomes increasingly easy, when the eyes are closed, to make a correct guess at the nature of the memory-image arising from the traces left by the act of sensing.

A good teacher can do much to help one in bringing up into consciousness the memory-images of what was merely sensed, not actually seen. Children, who are less self-conscious than their elders, respond particularly well to such a teacher's suggestions and encouragements. For example, a child is shown some object, say a domino, or a printed letter, or word, from a distance at which he cannot normally see it. He is told to take a flashing glance at it, then close his eyes and "reach up into the air for it." The child obeys the order quite literally, raises a hand, closes it on emptiness, then lowers it, opens it, looks into his palm and gives the correct answer, as though he were reading from notes.

After a certain amount of practice, the barrier between sensing and perceiving (always present in persons with defective vision) is so far lowered that unconscious vision (or the revival through memory of the traces left by sensing) gives place to conscious vision (or the perceiving of what is sensed in the same moment as it is sensed). In the early stages there is generally a rather long interval between the act of sensing and the act of perceiving. Several seconds may elapse before the person can say what he has seen. The psychological barrier interposed by strain between the eyes and the mind has been lowered, indeed, but not yet completely eliminated. But as time goes on the interval is progressively shortened, until at last sensing and perceiving take place as they normally should, almost simultaneously.

Techniques of Flashing

Flashing, like swinging, can be practiced during the activities of everyday life. For those whose vision is defective, the temptation to stare is always strong. Resist it, and acquire instead the habit of taking rapid glances at things, then averting or momentarily closing the eyes and remembering what was sensed. Billboards and shop-fronts provide excellent material on which to practice flashing, as one walks or is carried past them in car or bus. The mental attitude of one who is looking at the world in quick, brief flashes should be one of easy indifference. Just as, while swinging, one lets the world go by without making any effort to get to know it in detail, so, while flashing, one should rid one's mind of any over-anxious desire to see, and just be content to glance, first outwards at the physical object, then inwards at the memory-image of it. If the inward image corresponds with the outward object, as seen at a second and nearer glance, well and good. If it fails to correspond, but is merely a blur, that also is well and good. Nothing is so unfavorable to seeing as the competitive, prize-winning, test-passing spirit. Efforts on the part of the conscious "I" defeat their own object. It is when you stop trying to see that seeing comes to you.

Casual flashing should be supplemented by drills during periods specifically set aside for the purpose. The objects used in these drills should be fairly small, simple, clear-cut and familiar. Here, for example, are some effective procedures, in which use is made of a set of dominoes.

Relax the eyes by palming for a few moments; then pick up a

domino at random, hold it out at arm's length, pass the eyes across it in a quick glance and immediately close them. Even if the dots were not distinctly seen, it is probable that they were sensed, and that the sensing will have left a trace which can be revived as a memory-image. With the eyes still closed tell yourself what you remember to have made out of the upper half of the domino, then of the lower half. Open the eyes and, if necessary, bring the domino nearer for a verification of your guess. If the guess was right, well and good. If it was wrong, well and good. Take another domino and start again.

A more elaborate version of the same procedure is as follows. Take a dozen dominoes and stand them in a row along the edge of a table. Seat yourself in front of them at the limit of convenient seeing. Swing your eyes from left to right along the row, counting the dominoes as rapidly as you possibly can. (This sets the immobilized eyes and attention shifting at unaccustomed speed, and is a most salutary exercise in itself.) Then bring the eyes back to the first domino and, closing the lids, name the numbers in the upper and lower halves respectively. Open the eyes again and verify your guess. Then count the whole row once again and, glancing back to the second domino, flash, close, and name the numbers. Continue counting and flashing, until you reach the end of the line.

If your eyes are myopic, and it is hard to see at anything but short range, perform this drill for the first time within easy seeing distance; then move back and repeat. Familiarity with the dominoes will eliminate mental hazards and make the more distant seeing easier. It is possible in this way gradually to stretch the range of vision.

Where distant vision is easy, and difficulty is experienced only at the near point, this process should be reversed. Begin at some distance away; then move closer and go through the drill again.

Chapter 12

Shifting

Primarily designed to encourage mental and ocular mobility, the exercises described in the preceding chapters also serve, indirectly, to teach the art of central fixation. Having learned, by means of them, to keep the eyes and attention in constant movement, and being therefore less subject than before to the vice of mental and physical staring, we may safely proceed to a somewhat more direct approach to central fixation. Even now, however, the approach will not be completely direct. Before attempting to become fully conscious of the fact that we always see one small area more distinctly than all the rest, we shall be well advised to take some simple lessons in the art of continuous and concentrated looking. Swinging encourages the eyes and mind to make movements of considerable amplitude, and flashing teaches rapidity of motion and interpretative reaction. It is now necessary to teach ourselves small-scale shifting; for it is upon this small-scale shifting of eyes and mind that continuous, concentrated and attentive seeing depends. As I have pointed out before, the structure of the eyes and the nature of the mind are such that normal vision simply cannot take place without incessant small-scale shifting.

When regarding any object continuously and attentively, people with normal vision keep their eyes and attention shifting unconsciously in a series of almost imperceptibly small movements from point to point. People with defective vision, on the contrary, greatly reduce the number of such movements and tend to stare. It is therefore necessary for them to build up consciously the habit of small-scale shifting which they acquired unconsciously during childhood and subsequently lost.

Analytical Looking

The best way to do this is to learn to "look analytically" at any object you wish to consider with close attention. Do not stare; stop trying to see all parts of the object equally clearly at the same time. Instead, deliberately tell yourself to see it piecemeal, sensing and perceiving, one at a time, all the more significant parts of which it is composed.

For example, when looking at a house, note the number of windows, chimneys and doors. Follow with your eyes the outline of its silhouette against the sky. Let your glance run horizontally along the line of the eaves, and vertically up and down the wall spaces between the windows. And so on.

This kind of analytical looking is recommended in all systems designed to improve the powers of memory and concentration. It enables the looker to form clear mental concepts of what he has seen. Instead of staring and vaguely recording an image, to which he gives the name of "house," the person who does his looking analytically will be able to tell you a number of interesting and significant facts about that house—that it has, let us say, four windows and a front door on the ground floor and five windows above, one chimney at either end, and a tiled roof. This detailed knowledge of the house, which is the result of analytical looking, will tend to improve the vision of the same object when regarded on subsequent occasions. For we see most clearly things which are familiar; and an increase in our conceptual knowledge of an object always tends to facilitate the sensing of that object in the future. Thus we see that analytical looking not merely improves vision there and then, by compelling the eyes and mind to shift continuously from point to point; it also helps to improve vision at all later dates, by increasing our conceptual knowledge of the object regarded, and so making it seem more familiar and therefore easier to sense and perceive.

The process of analytical looking can be profitably applied even to such extremely familiar objects as letters, numerals, advertising slogans and the faces of one's relatives and friends. However well we may think we know such things, we shall almost certainly find, if we take to looking at them analytically, that we can get to know them a good deal better. When you look at letters or numerals, run the eyes over their outlines; observe the shapes of the pieces of background in contact with them, or included within them; count the number of corners on a block capital letter or large numeral. If you do this, the eyes and attention will be forced to do a great deal of small-scale shifting, which will improve the vision; and at the same time you will learn a great many hitherto unrecognized facts, the knowledge of which will help you to do a better and more rapid job of sensing on future occasions.

Persons with defective sight tend to do some of the intensest and most rigid staring when conversing with their fellow humans. Faces are very important to us, since it is by observing their changes of expression that we acquire much of our most valuable information about the thoughts, feelings and dispositions of those with whom we come in contact. To obtain this information people with defective vision make the most strenuous efforts to see the faces of those who surround them. In other words, they stare harder than usual. The result is discomfort and embarrassment for the persons stared at, and poorer vision for the starer. The remedy is analytical looking. Do not stare at faces, in the vain hope of seeing every part of them as clearly as every other part. Instead, shift the regard rapidly over the face you are looking at—from eye to eye, from ear to ear, from mouth to forehead. You will see the details of the face and its expression more clearly; and at the same time, to the person you are looking at, you will not seem to be staring—merely looking in a relaxed and easy way, with eyes to which your rapid, small-scale shifting imparts the brilliancy and sparkle of mobility.

Habits of continuous and small-scale shifting should be deliberately cultivated on all occasions during the day's activities when there is need for prolonged and concentrated seeing, either at the near or the far point. There are also certain drills, which it is well to practice during periods especially set aside for the purpose.

Teachers of the art of seeing have devised a considerable number of shifting drills, all of them effective if properly practiced. In this place I shall mention only one—a particularly good example of its kind—developed by Mrs. Margaret D. Corbett, and described in her book, *How to Improve Your Eyes.*

The only piece of material needed for the practice of this drill is a sheet from one of those large, tear-off calendars, in which the current month is printed in large type across the upper part of the page, while the previous and succeeding months appear below in much smaller type. Inasmuch as it offers type of different sizes, such a sheet possesses most of the advantages of the graduated Snellen Chart, used by oculists for testing vision. Inasmuch as a row of consecutive numbers presents no mental hazards, it possesses none of the Snellen Chart's disadvantages—unfamiliarity and the intent to confuse and deceive, almost always present in the minds of those who design such devices for testing vision. Since our aim is not to test, but to improve sight, we shall do well to make use of the most familiar, and therefore the most visible and confidence-creating objects upon which to exercise. A calendar fulfills these conditions perfectly, and possesses the further merit of not having the unpleasant associations of the Snellen Chart. Most children and many adults dislike having their eyes examined and become so nervous, when tested, that they see much worse than at ordinary times. Consequently, the Snellen Chart is apt to be surrounded, for them, by a kind of aura of disagreeableness, which makes it one of the least visible of objects. That is why Snellen Charts should be used for visual self-education only by those to whom they are emotionally neutral, and only when the user is completely familiar with every line of graduated type, from the big two-hundred-foot letter at the top to the tiny ten-foot letters at the bottom of the card. If these conditions are not fulfilled, the Snellen Chart may easily prove a source of anxiety and strain. A good teacher will note his pupil's tendency towards strain and take steps to prevent it from coming to a head. Consequently, it is always safe for a good teacher to make use of the Snellen Chart as an instrument of visual training. The self-instructed will do better to start, at any rate, with other training material.

The Calendar Drill

In working with the calendar we begin by loosening up the staring mind and eyes by means of a procedure very similar to that employed in one of the domino drills. Hang the calendar on a wall, at a level with your eyes when you are seated. See that the sheet is well illuminated, either by direct or reflected sunlight, or (if the sun is not shining) by ordinary daylight or a strong lamp. Draw up a chair, and sit down in front of it, at a point from which the larger print can be seen without difficulty. Palm the eyes for a little, then set to work in the following way.

Turn the head to the left, as though you were glancing over your shoulder; then swing it back, gently and not too fast, until the eyes rest on the figure "one" of the large-type calendar. Take note of the figure, then close the eyes and breathe deeply and easily, swinging your head a little as you do so, in order to keep the rhythm of your movement unbroken. After a few seconds turn to look over the right shoulder, reopen the eyes and swing them back until they rest on the figure "two." Close again as before, turn to the left and swing back to the "three." And so on.

When swinging down the line towards the selected figure, always let the regard travel in the white space immediately below the print. A blank surface, such as the background to printed words or numerals, presents no difficulties to the interpreting mind and cannot, therefore, be a source of strain. Consequently, when the regard is made to move along the white space immediately under the line of type, the mind reaches its objective in a state of relaxation—with the result that the attention and the eyes can do their work of rapid, small-scale shifting and central fixation under the best possible conditions.

After going through the whole month, or as much of it as you have time for, palm the eyes for a little, and proceed to the next phase of the drill. As this procedure demands a more attentive kind of looking than the preceding exercise, you will find yourself more than ordinarily tempted to hold your breath. Resist the temptation and, during all the time you are at practice, keep the breathing going consciously at a little more than its average amplitude.

Glance at the figure "one" in the large-type calendar, then drop the eyes to the corresponding figure in the small-type calendar at the bottom of the sheet to the left. Look at it only for a moment, then close and relax for a few seconds. Open the eyes once more on the figure "one" in the large-type calendar, and drop to the "one" in the small-type calendar to the right. Close the eyes again in an easy, relaxed way, and keep the breathing going. Then reopen—this time on the large "two." Drop to the small "two" on the left. Close, breathe, reopen on the large "two," and drop to the small "two" on the right. Close again, breathe, and continue with the other numbers in the same way, either to the end of the month or, if the drill seems tiring, to the end of the first week or fortnight.

At first there may be difficulty in seeing the small-type numerals. If there is, do not linger over them, or make an effort to see them. Instead of that, adopt the technique described in the chapter on flashing. Glance easily and unconcernedly at the small number; then, in the brief period during which the eyes are closed, note whether there is any memory-image of it. You will be aided in this search for the indistinct image of the smaller numeral by your clearer memory of the larger, but otherwise exactly similar numeral. Knowing just what it is you should have seen, you will soon find yourself seeing it—at first, perhaps, unconsciously, as the memory-image of something only dimly sensed; then consciously and with increasing clarity at the moment of sensing.

After an interval of palming, proceed to the next phase of the drill. With eyes closed, think of any number between one and thirty-one. Let us assume that you begin by thinking of the number "seventeen." Open the eyes and, as quickly as you possibly can, locate "seventeen," first on the large-type calendar, then on the small calendar on the left. Close and breathe. Then reopen on the large "seventeen" and drop to the corresponding small number on the right. Close once more, breathe, think of another number, and go through the same procedure. After ten or a dozen repetitions, you will be ready to go on to the next phase.

In this drill we return to the small-scale shift, which we learn to practice systematically, with a very short rhythmic swing, on such objects as letters and numerals. Look at the large "one." Pay attention first to the top of the numeral, then to the base; then shift the eyes and mind once more to the top and again to the base. Up and down, up and down, two or three times. When you have done this, close the eyes in a relaxed way and breathe deeply but gently. Then reopen the eyes and repeat the procedure on the large "two." After going through half the month in this way, drop to one of the small-type calendars and begin again, drawing your chair a little nearer, if necessary.

The procedure should be varied by sometimes making the shift horizontally, swinging from one side of the numeral to the other side, instead of up and down, in a vertical direction. Furthermore, do not confine yourself exclusively to the numerals. Work also on letters— the SUN., MON., TUES., and so on, of the abbreviated days of the week. Do the small-scale swinging shift from top to bottom of these letters, and from side to side, and, in the case of the broader and more angular ones, from corner to corner, diagonally. Letters and numerals are among the most familiar objects in our artificial world, and among the objects which it is most important for us to see clearly. It is therefore especially desirable that we should acquire the habit of small-scale shifting when we regard these objects. Conscious practice of the swinging shift, just described, will end by building up a beneficent automatism. Whenever we regard a letter or numeral, we shall tend, unconsciously and automatically, to practice the small-scale shift, which compels the eyes and mind to do their work by central fixation and, in this way, improves our sensing, our perceiving and that end-product of sensing and perceiving, our vision. In the chapters dealing with the mental side of seeing, I shall describe procedures in which this technique of the small-scale swinging shift is combined with techniques for the development of memory and imagination, and so rendered still more valuable. But even in its simple form, as I have described it in the preceding paragraphs, the procedure is remarkably effective. While practicing these calendar drills you will constantly be struck by the way in which vision improves when the small-scale swinging shift is made use of. The numeral or letter, which appeared so dim and hazy, when you first looked at it, will come up into clear definition as you shift your attention a few times from top to base, or from side to side. The same technique should be carried over into the ordinary activities of life. When confronted by letters or numerals you cannot clearly distinguish, try the small-scale swinging shift on them, and they will tend to brighten and grow more definite.

This particular kind of shifting is simply analytical looking with a regular rhythm. Regular rhythmic movement is always relaxing, even when repeated only a few times, and this is why the small-scale swinging shift is so effective in promoting good vision. It is, unfortunately, impracticable to use this swinging shift on all classes of objects. On such small, clearly demarcated and thoroughly familiar objects as numerals and letters it is easy to perform the swinging shift. But where the object is large, relatively unfamiliar, indeterminate or in motion, it is not feasible, for the simple reason that either there are no known and definite landmarks, no clearly outlined boundaries, between which to do the repeated shift, or, if there are such landmarks and boundaries, the area covered by the eyes, as they shift back and forth from one to the other, will be so small in comparison with the total area of the object that an improved knowledge of that area will not necessarily give an improved knowledge of the whole. Consequently, in the case of large, indeterminate and unfamiliar objects, the best technique of looking remains the rapid analytical regard, without repetitive rhythm. The effectiveness of this analytical regard may be enhanced by counting the salient features of the object. If there are many such features, do not try to count them with pedantic accuracy. What is important is not to know the correct total, but to make the attention realize that large numbers of such features exist and must be noted. So count only the first three or four; then skim over the rest and make a guess at the total, not caring whether your guess is correct or not. Your goal is to see more clearly, and that goal will have been achieved, if the pretence at counting stimulates the eyes and attention to do their work of rapid, small-scale shifting, in act after act of central fixation.

And now, having learned the means whereby central fixation may be rendered habitual and automatic, let us take the last step in this long series of exercises, and make ourselves fully conscious of the fact that we see best only a small part of what we are looking at. For many of those who have undertaken the exercises, there will be no need to take this step, for the good reason that they have already acquired that awareness. It is hard to look at things analytically, or to practice the small-scale swinging shift without discovering the fact of central fixation.

Those who have not yet observed the phenomenon may now, without any serious risk of strain or effort, take the following steps to convince themselves of its regular occurrence. Hold up the forefingers of either hand about two feet from the face and about eighteen inches apart. Look first at the right forefinger. It will be seen more distinctly than the left, which appears at the extreme edge of the field of vision. Now turn the head and pay attention to the left finger, which will at once be seen more clearly than the right. Now bring the fingers closer together. Look from one to the other when they are a foot apart, then six inches, then three inches, then one inch, then when they are actually touching. In all cases the finger regarded by the eyes and attended to by the mind will be seen more distinctly than the other.

Repeat the same process on a letter—say a large E from a front-page newspaper headline. Pay attention first to the top bar of the E, and notice that it seems clearer and blacker than the other two bars. Then shift attention to the bottom bar, and note how *that* is now the clearest of the three. Do the same with the middle bar. Next out a smaller E from some less strident headline and repeat the process. You will find, if the eyes and mind have lost their old bad habit of staring, that even in the smaller letter there is a perceptible difference in distinctness between the bar which is actually being attended to and the bars which are not being attended to. As time goes on it will be possible to observe differences in distinctness between the upper and lower part even of a small twelve-point or eight-point letter. The more perfect the sight, the smaller the area which can be seen with maximum distinctness.

To confirm the fact of central fixation, one may reverse the process described above and do one's best to see every part of a large letter, or every feature of a friend's face, equally clearly at the same time. The result will be an almost immediate sense of strain and a lowering of vision. One cannot with impunity attempt to do the physically and psychologically impossible. But that, precisely, is what the person with defective sight is perpetually doing when he peers with such an anxious intentness at the world around him. Once you have convinced yourself experimentally of this fact, and of the other, complementary fact that good vision comes only when the eyes and mind make innumerable successive acts of central fixation, you will never again be tempted to stare, to strain, to try hard to see. Vision is not won by making an effort to get it; it comes to those who have learned to put their minds and eyes into a state of alert passivity, of dynamic relaxation.

Chapter 13

The Mental Side of Seeing

The eyes provide us with the visual sense impressions, which are the raw materials of sight. The mind takes these raw materials and works them up into the finished product—normal vision of external objects.

When sight is subnormal, the defect may be due to causes belonging to one or other of two main categories, physical and mental. The eyes, or the nervous system connected with them, may suffer accidental injury, or be affected by disease—in which case the supply of the raw materials of vision will be cut off at the source. Alternatively, the efficiency of the mind, as the interpreter of crude *sensa,* may be impaired owing to any one of a great number of possible psychological maladjustments. When this happens, the efficiency of the eye as a sensing apparatus is also impaired; for the human mind-body is a single unit, and psychological malfunctioning is reflected in physiological malfunctioning. With the impairment of the physiological functioning of the eye, the quality of the raw materials which it furnishes falls off; and this in turn increases the inefficiency of the mind as a worker-up of such materials.

Orthodox ophthalmologists are content to palliate the symptoms of poor sight by means of "those valuable crutches," artificial lenses. They work only on the sensing eye and ignore completely the selecting, perceiving and seeing mind. It is a case of *Hamlet* without the Prince of Denmark. Obviously and on the face of it, any rational, any genuinely aetiological treatment of defective vision must take account of the mental side of seeing. In the method of visual re-education, developed by Dr. W.H. Bates and his followers, due attention is paid not merely to the provider of raw materials, but also to the producer of the finished article.

Of the psychological factors which prevent the mind from doing a good job of interpretation, some are closely related to the process of perceiving and seeing, while others are not. In the latter category we must place all those negative emotions which are so fruitful a source of malfunctioning and, finally, of organic disease in every part of the body, including the eyes. To the former belong certain negative emotions specifically related to the act of seeing, and certain malfunctionings of the memory and imagination—malfunctionings which lower the mind's efficiency as an interpreter of *sensa*.

To treat of the methods by which negative emotions may be avoided or dispelled is beyond the scope of this little book. I can only repeat in different words what was said in the opening section. When the conscious "I" is afflicted to excess by such emotions as fear, anger, worry, grief, envy, ambition, the mind and body are likely to suffer. One of the important psycho-physical functions most commonly impaired is that of vision. Negative emotions impair vision, partly through direct action upon the nervous, glandular and circulatory systems, partly by lowering the efficiency of the mind. It is literally true that people become "blind with rage"; that fear may make the world "go black" or "swim before the eyes"; that worry can be so "numbing" that people cease to be able to see or hear properly, and are therefore frequently involved in serious accidents. Nor are the effects of such negative emotions merely transient and temporary. If they are intense enough and sufficiently protracted, negative feelings such as worry, disappointed love and competitiveness, can produce in their victim serious organic derangements—for example, gastric ulcer, tuberculosis and coronary disease. They can also produce lasting malfunctioning of the seeing organs, mental and physical—malfunctioning that manifests itself in mental strain, nervous muscular tension and errors of refraction. Anybody who wants normal vision should therefore do everything possible to avoid or get rid of these pernicious negative emotions, and in the meanwhile should learn the art of seeing, by means of which the disastrous effects of such emotions upon the eyes and mind can be completely or partially undone.

This seems to be all that can be usefully said, in this place at any rate, about those mental obstacles to normal vision, which are not immediately connected with the act of seeing. For a full discussion of negative emotions, and for methods of dealing with them, one must turn to the psychiatrists, the moralists and the writers on ascetical and mystical religion. In a brief introduction to the art of seeing, I can only mention the problem and pass on.

We have now to consider those mental obstacles to normal vision which are intimately bound up with the actual seeing process. Certain negative emotions, habitually associated with the act of seeing by people with subnormal vision, have already been discussed. Thus, I have described the fear of light, and the means by which that fear may be cast out. I have also mentioned that greed for vision, that over-anxiety to see too much too well, which results in misdirection of attention and in mental and physical staring; and I have dwelled at great length on the procedures by means of which these bad habits may be changed, and the undesirable emotions, responsible for them, dispelled.

We have now to consider another fear, intimately connected in the minds of those suffering from defective vision with the act of seeing, and responsible in some degree for the perpetuation of visual malfunctioning. I refer to the fear of not seeing properly.

Let us trace the genealogy of this fear. The art of seeing in a normal and natural way is acquired unconsciously during infancy and childhood. Then, owing to physical disease or, more often to mental strain, good seeing habits are lost; normal and natural functioning is replaced by abnormal and unnatural functioning; the mind loses its efficiency as an interpreter, the physical conformation of the eye is distorted and the net result is that vision is impaired. From subnormal vision there springs, in most cases, a certain chronic apprehension. The person who is used to seeing badly is afraid that he will see badly next time. In the minds of many afflicted men and women this fearful anticipation amounts to a fixed, intense, pessimistic *conviction* that for them normal seeing is henceforth impossible.

Such an attitude is paralyzing to the minds and eyes of those who entertain it. They go into every new seeing situation afraid that they won't see, or even convinced in advance that they can't see. The result, not unnaturally, is that they don't see. Positive faith enables a man to move mountains. Conversely, negative faith can prevent him from lifting a straw.

In seeing, as in all other activities of mind and mind-body, it is essential, if we are to do our work adequately, that we should cultivate an attitude of confidence combined with indifference—confidence in our capacity to do the job, and indifference to possible failure. We must feel sure that we can succeed some time, if we use the proper means and exercise sufficient patience; and we must not feel disappointed or annoyed if in fact we don't succeed this particular time.

Confidence untempered by indifference may be almost as disastrous as the lack of confidence; for if we feel sure that we are going to succeed, and are distressed and affronted every time we fail, confidence will only be a source of negative emotions, which will in their turn increase the probability of failure.

For the person whose sight is subnormal, the correct mental attitude may be expressed in some such words as these. "I know theoretically that defective vision can be improved. I feel certain that, if I learn the art of seeing, I can improve my own defective vision. I am practicing the art of seeing as I look now, and it is likely that I shall see better than I did; but if I don't see as well as I hope, I shall not feel wretched or aggrieved, but go on, until better vision comes to me."

Chapter 14

Memory and Imagination

The capacity for perception depends, as I have shown in an earlier chapter, upon the amount, the kind and the availability of past experiences. But past experiences exist for us only in the memory. Therefore it is true to say that perception depends upon memory.

Closely related to memory is imagination, which is the power of recombining memories in novel ways, so as to make mental constructions different from anything actually experienced in the past. The mind's ability to interpret *sensa* is affected by the imagination as well as the memory.

The extent to which perception and, consequently, vision are dependent upon memory and imagination is a matter of everyday experience. We see familiar things more clearly than we see objects about which we have no stock of memories. And when under emotional stress or excitement our imagination is more than ordinarily active, it often happens that we interpret *sensa* as manifestations of the objects with which our imagination is busy, rather than as manifestation of the objects actually present in the external world. The old seamstress, who cannot read without glasses, can see to thread her needle with the naked eye. Why? Because she is more familiar with needles than with print.

In the book he is reading, a person with normal vision comes upon a strange, polysyllabic, technical word, or a phrase in some foreign language of which he is ignorant. The letters of which these words are composed are precisely similar to those in which the rest of the book is printed; and yet this person finds it definitely harder to see them. Why? Because the rest of the book is in plain English, while the illegible words are in German, shall we say, or Russian, or the Greco-Latin jargon of one of the sciences.

A man who can work all day at the office without undue fatigue of the eyes, is worn out by an hour at a museum, and comes home with a splitting headache. Why? Because at the office he is following a regular routine and looking at words and figures, the like of which he looks at every day; whereas in the museum everything is strange, novel and outlandish.

Or take the case of the lady who is terrified of snakes, and who mistakes what to everyone else is obviously a length of rubber tubing for an enormous viper. Her vision, as tested on the Snellen chart, is normal. Why, then, does she see what isn't there? Because her imagination had been in the habit of using old memories of snakes to construct alarming images of the creatures, and because under the influence of her imagination her mind misinterpreted the *sensa* connected with the rubber tubing in such a way that she vividly "saw" a viper.

Such examples which could be multiplied almost indefinitely leave no doubt that perception and therefore vision depend upon memory and to a lesser degree imagination. We see best the things about which, or the likes of which, we have a good stock of memories. And the more accurate these memories are, the more thoroughgoing and analytical the knowledge they embody, the better (all other things being equal) will be the vision. Indeed, the vision may be better, even when other things are not equal. Thus, the veteran microscopist may have worse sight, as measured on the Snellen chart, than the first-year undergraduate whom he is instructing. Nevertheless, when he looks through his instrument he will be able, thanks to his accurate memories of similar objects, to see the slide much more clearly than the novice can.

The truth that perception and vision are largely dependent upon past experiences, as recorded by the memory, has been recognized for centuries. But, so far as I am aware, the first person ever to pay any serious thought to what I may call the utilitarian and therapeutic corollaries of this truth was Dr. W.H. Bates. He it was who first asked the question: "How can this dependence of perception and vision upon memory and, to a lesser degree, imagination be exploited so as to improve people's sight?" And having asked the question, he did not rest until he had found a number of simple and practical answers. His followers have been working for many years on the same problem, and they too have produced their quota of devices for improving vision by working on the memory and imagination. Here, I shall give an account of some of the more effective of these procedures. But first a few more words about certain significant characteristics of that most mysterious mental activity, remembering.

Perhaps the most important fact about memory in its relation to perception and vision is that it will not work well under strain. Everyone is familiar with the experience of forgetting a name, straining to recapture it and ignominiously failing. Then, if one is wise, one will stop trying to remember and allow the mind to sink into a condition of alert passivity; the chances are that the name will come bobbing up into consciousness of its own accord. Memory works best, it would seem, when the mind is in a state of dynamic relaxation.

Experience has taught the great majority of people that there is a correlation between good memory and dynamic relaxation of mind—a condition which always tends to be accompanied by dynamic relaxation of the body as well.

They have never formulated the fact explicitly to themselves; but they know it unconsciously, or to be more precise they consistently act as though they knew it unconsciously. When they try to remember something, they instinctively "let go," because they have learned, in the course of innumerable repetitions of the act of remembering that the condition of "letting go" is the most favorable for good memory. Now, this habit of "letting go" in order to remember persists, in many cases, even when bad habits of mental and physical tension have been built up in relation to other activities, such as seeing. Consequently it often happens that, when people start remembering, they automatically and unconsciously put themselves into that condition of dynamic mental relaxation, which is propitious not only for memory but also for vision. This would seem to be the explanation of the fact (first observed, so far as I know, by Dr. Bates, but easily observable by anyone who is ready to fulfill the necessary conditions) that the simple act of remembering something clearly and distinctly brings an immediate improvement of vision.

In some cases of defective vision the state of mental and physical tension is so extreme that the sufferers have lost the habit of "letting go," even when remembering. The result is that they have the greatest difficulty in recalling anything. Experienced teachers of the Bates Method have told me of pupils who came to them incapable of remembering ten seconds after the event whether they had been looking at letters, numerals or pictures. As soon as the eyes and mind had been somewhat relaxed by means of palming, sunning, swinging and shifting, the power to remember returned. The imperfect vision and the state of virtual imbecility into which the inability to remember had plunged these unfortunate people were due to the same fundamental cause—improper functioning, associated with a high degree of mental and nervous muscular strain.

Fortunately such cases are not common; and the majority of those who suffer from defects of vision due to or aggravated by mental and physical strain still preserve the good habit acquired unconsciously through the teachings of everyday experience, of "letting go" whenever they make an act of remembering. That is why it is possible with most individuals to make use of memory as an aid to mind-body relaxation and, through mind-body relaxation, to vision. A person with defective sight looks, let us say, at a printed letter and fails to see it distinctly. If he closes his eyes, "lets go" and remembers something which it is easy for him to remember—remembers it clearly and distinctly—he will find on reopening his eyes that his vision has perceptibly improved.

Because it is impossible to remember anything clearly without "letting go," improvement of vision will follow the act of remembering any object or episode, even one totally unconnected with the thing which at the moment it is desired to see. But if the memory is actually of this thing, or of some similar thing seen in the past, then the act of remembering will be doubly effective in improving vision; for it will result not only in producing a beneficent relaxation of the mind-body, but also in an increased familiarity with the object under consideration. But we see most clearly those things with which we are most familiar. Consequently, any procedure which makes us more familiar with the object we are trying to see makes it easier for us to see it. But every act of remembering that object or another one like it increases our familiarity with it and so improves our vision of it. It is because of this fact that several of the most important memory and imagination drills are concerned with the detailed remembering or visualizing of the letters and figures which we are so constantly being called upon to see, both at the near point and in the distance.

In the light of these preliminary explanations it will be easy, I hope, for the reader to understand the various procedures now to be described.

Memory as an Aid to Vision

The value of what I have called analytical looking can be enhanced by supplementing this procedure with deliberate acts of memory. Look at objects in the way described in an earlier chapter—shifting the attention rapidly from point to point, following the outlines and counting the salient features of what you are looking at. Then close your eyes, "let go" and conjure up the clearest possible memory-image of what you have just seen. Reopen the eyes, compare this image with the reality, and repeat the process of analytical looking. Close the eyes, and once more evoke the memory-image of what you have seen. After a few repetitions there will be an improvement in the clarity and accuracy both of the memory-image and of the visual image recorded when the eyes are open.

It is a good thing to practice these acts of analytical looking and remembering in relation to the objects of one's everyday environment, such as the furniture of the rooms in which one lives and works, the shops and billboards, trees and houses of the streets one ordinarily frequents. This will have three good results: it will break up the habit of staring and encourage central fixation; it will compel the mind to put itself into the state of alert passivity, of dynamic relaxation, which alone is conducive to accurate remembering, and incidentally, to clear vision; and it will greatly increase the mind's knowledge of and familiarity with the objects it must see most frequently, and by doing so will greatly facilitate the task of seeing these objects.

Nor is this all. The procedure outlined above is also beneficial inasmuch as it teaches a proper coordination between the mind and its sensing apparatus. Too many of us spend altogether too much of our time looking at one thing and thinking of another—seeing just enough to avoid running into trees or under buses, but at the same time daydreaming so much that if anyone were to ask us what we had seen, we should find it almost impossible to answer for the good reason that though we had sensed a great deal, we had consciously perceived almost nothing. This dissociation of the mind from its eyes is a fruitful cause of impairment of vision, particularly when, as is very frequently the case, the daydreaming person sits with open eyes, staring fixedly and unblinkingly at one point. If you must daydream, close your eyes, and with your inward vision consciously follow the wish-fulfilling episodes fabricated by the imagination. Similarly, when engaged in logical thought, do not stare at some external object unconnected with the problem under consideration. If the eyes are kept open, use them to do something relevant to the intellectual processes going on within the mind. For example, write notes which the eyes can read, or draw diagrams for them to study. Alternatively, if the eyes are kept closed, resist the temptation of immobilizing them—a temptation which is always strong when one is making an effort at mental concentration. Let the inward eye travel over imaginary words, diagrams or other constructions relevant to the thought process which is taking place. The aim at all times should be to prevent the occurrence of dissociations between mind and sensing apparatus. When the eyes are open, make a point of seeing and of being conscious of what you see. When you don't want to see, but to dream or think, make a point of associating the eyes with your dreaming or thinking. By allowing the mind to go one way and the eyes another, you run the risk of impairing your vision, which is a product of the cooperation between a physical sensing apparatus and a selecting and perceiving intelligence.

Improving the Memory of Letters

For good as well as for evil, reading has now become one of the principal occupations of civilized humanity. Inability to read easily, whether at the near point or at a distance, is a serious handicap in the contemporary world. The art of reading will be discussed at length in one of the later chapters of this book. Here I shall describe certain procedures by means of which the forces of memory and imagination can be mobilized for the improvement of our vision of those basic constituents of all literature and science, the twenty-six letters of the alphabet and the ten numerals.

One of the curious facts discovered by teachers who undertake the re-education of sufferers from defective vision is that very large numbers of people do not have a clear mental image of the letters of the alphabet. Capitals, it is true, are familiar to almost everyone—perhaps because it is upon capital letters that the young child first practices the art of reading. But lower case letters, though looked at hundreds of times each day, are so imperfectly known that many persons find it hard to reproduce them exactly, or to recognize a given letter from it description in words. This widespread ignorance of the forms of letters bears eloquent witness to the dissociation between eyes and mind described in the preceding paragraphs.

In this matter of reading, we are such greedy end-gainers that we neglect to consider not merely the psycho-physical means whereby we may accomplish the task most effectively, but also the external, objective means upon which the whole process of reading depends, namely the letters of the alphabet. There can be no improvement in our ability to read until we have made ourselves thoroughly familiar with the letters of which all reading matter is composed. Here again it is a question of combining analytical looking with acts of remembering.

Examine a letter, not with a fixed stare, but easily and with a rapid shift of the attention from one point to another. Close the eyes, "let go" and evoke the memory-image of what you have seen. Reopen the eyes, and check the accuracy of your memory. Repeat the process until the memory-image is thoroughly accurate, distinct and clear. Do the same with all the letters—and, of course, all the numerals as well. The exercise may be repeated occasionally, even when you think you know all the letters perfectly. Memory can always be improved; besides, the act of remembering brings relaxation, and this relaxation, combined with the heightened familiarity which comes of better memory, will always tend to improve the vision.

When looking at letters, with the aim of familiarizing oneself with their forms, it is well to pay attention, not only to the black print, but also and above all to the white background immediately surrounding the letters and included within them. These areas of whiteness around and within letters and numerals have curious and striking shapes, which the mind enjoys getting to know and, because of its interest in them, remembers easily. At the same time, there is less possibility of mental strain involved in considering the blank background than in considering the black marks upon that background. It is often easier to see a letter when it is regarded as an interruption to the whiteness of the paper than when it is looked at without conscious reference to the background, merely as a pattern of straight and curved black lines.

This process of familiarizing oneself with letters, by analytical looking and remembering, may profitably be supplemented by a drill involving the systematic use of imagination. Examine the letter as before, paying attention to the shapes of the background around and within it. Then close the eyes, "let go," evoke a memory-image of the letter and then deliberately imagine that the white background around and within it is whiter than it was actually seen to be—as white as snow or sunlit cloud or porcelain.

Reopen the eyes and look again at the letter, shifting as before from background-shape to background-shape, and trying to see these shapes as white as you imagined them with your eyes shut. In a little while you will find that you can, without difficulty, create this beneficent illusion. When you succeed in doing so the black of the printer's ink will seem blacker by contrast, and there will be a perceptible improvement in vision.

Sometimes, by way of change, one may use the imagination in an analogous way upon the black letter itself. Seated before the calendar, pay attention first to the top of a numeral or letter, then to the base (or first to the left side and then to the right). After a few repetitions, close the eyes, "let go" and continue to do the same thing to your memory-image of the numeral or letter. Then, in imagination, apply two spots of intenser blackness, one to the top and the other to the base, or one on the left and the other on the right. If you find it helpful, imagine yourself applying these spots with a fine paint brush impregnated with India ink.

Shift from one blacker spot to the other several times; then open the eyes and try to see the same blacker spots at the top and base, or on the left and right sides, of the real letter. This will not be difficult, because owing to central fixation you actually will see that part of the letter or numeral which you are attending to more clearly than the rest. But imagine the spots to be even blacker than central fixation warrants. When you succeed in doing this the whole letter will seem blacker than before, and will therefore be seen more clearly and remembered more distinctly for future reference.

These two procedures—shifting first in imagination, then in reality, from one area of whiter-than-acutal whiteness to another area of whiter-than-actual whiteness, and from one more intensely black dot to another more intensely black dot at the opposite end of the letter—are particularly helpful in improving vision, and should be used (in conjunction, if possible, with palming and sunning) whenever the print of a book, or a distant billboard or notice, shows signs of blurring.

Certain other procedures involving imagination have also proved their worth in visual education. The first three closely resemble the small-scale swinging shift—indeed, *are* swinging shifts, but of an exclusively mental kind.

Imagine yourself seated at a writing table, with a pad of thick white notepaper before you. Still in imagination, take a pen or a fine paint brush, dip it in India ink, and at the center of the first sheet of paper make a round black dot. Now pay attention to the white background immediately adjoining the right side of the dot, then to that immediately adjoining the left, and repeat, swinging rhythmically back and forth. As in reality, the imaginary dot will appear to move to the left, when you shift attention to the right. Conversely, the dot will appear to move to the right, when you shift attention to the left.

The following variant on the single dot may be used if desired. On another sheet of imaginary paper inscribe two dots, about four inches apart, and between them, but about an inch below them, a circle of about half an inch in diameter. Imagine this circle very black, and the white space within it intensely white. Then shift the inward eye from the dot on the right, to the dot on the left, and repeat the action rhythmically. The movement of the circle will be in the opposite direction to that of the attention.

Next, in your imagination, take another sheet of paper and trace upon it a giant colon, composed of two big dots about half an inch apart, and next to it, half an inch to the right, a semicolon of the same proportions. Now, shift the attention from the upper dot of the colon to the upper dot of the semicolon; then down to the comma of the semicolon; then, left, to the lower dot of the colon; and from that, vertically, to the upper dot. Repeat this rhythmic shifting round and round the square composed by the three round dots and the comma. As the mind's eye travels to the right, the constellation of punctuation marks will appear to move to the left; as the attention descends it will seem to go up; as it shifts to the left, the apparent movement will be to the right; and as it moves up to its original starting point, the dots will seem to descend.

These three procedures combine the merits of the small-scale swinging shift with those of the imagination drill. The mind has to relax enough to be able to mobilize its memory-images of punctuation marks, and combine them into simple patterns, while the attention (and consequently the physical eyes) is made to cultivate the sight-producing habit of the small-scale swinging shift—a shift which, in the third procedure, becomes a rhythmic version of the analytical regard.

The following procedure was devised by a Spanish follower of Dr. Bates, and the author of a book and various articles on the method, Dr. R. Arnau.

It is a kind of imaginary shifting swing—but a shifting swing with a difference, inasmuch as it seems to involve the physical apparatus of accommodation in ways which the ordinary swinging shift does not.

Imagine yourself holding between the thumb and forefinger a ring of stout rubber or wire, sufficiently rigid to retain its circular shape when not interfered with, but sufficiently elastic to assume when squeezed the form of an ellipse. Close the lids, and regard this imaginary ring, running the inward eye all around it. Then, with your imaginary hand, gently squeeze the ring laterally, so that it is deformed into an ellipse with the long axis running vertically. Look at this ellipse for a moment, then relax the pressure of your hand and allow the ring to return to its circular form. Now, shift the position of the thumb and forefinger from the sides of the ring to the top and bottom, and squeeze. The ring will be distorted into an ellipse with the long axis running horizontally. Relax the pressure, watch the ellipse retransform itself into a circle, shift the position of thumb and forefinger to the sides of the ring and repeat the whole procedure ten or fifteen times, rhythmically. Exactly what happens, physiologically, as one watches, in imagination, the successive transformations of circle into vertically orientated ellipse, vertically orientated ellipse into circle, circle into horizontally orientated ellipse, and horizontally orientated ellipse into circle, it is hard to say. But there can be no doubt, from the sensations one feels in and around the eye, that considerable muscular adjustments and readjustments are continually taking place, as one goes through this cycle of visualizations. Subjectively, these sensations seem to be the same as those experienced when one shifts the attention rapidly from the distance to a point very near the eyes and back again. Why the apparatus of accommodation should come into play under these conditions it is not easy to understand. But the fact remains that it seems to do so. It is found empirically that this drill, while valuable in all forms of visual defect, is particularly useful in cases of myopia.

Another excellent procedure, which is simultaneously an exercise in mind-body coordination, an imagination drill, and a small-scale shift, is "nose-writing." Sitting down comfortably in an easy chair, close your eyes and imagine that you have a good long pencil attached to the end of your nose. (Lovers of Edward Lear will remember his pictures of the "Dong.") Equipped with this instrument, move your head and neck so as to write with your protracted nose upon an imaginary sheet of paper (or, if the pencil is thought of as being white, on an imaginary blackboard) eight or nine inches in front of your face. Begin by drawing a good-sized circle. Since your control over the movements of the head and neck is less perfect than your control of the hand, this circle will certainly look a bit angular and lopsided to the eyes of your imagination. Go over it half a dozen times, round and round, until the thickened circumference comes to look presentable. Then draw a line from the top of your circle to the bottom, and go over it six times. Draw another line at right angles to the first and go over that in the same way. Your circle will now contain a St. George's Cross, by drawing two diagonals, and finish off by jabbing with your imaginary pencil at the central meeting-place of the four lines.

Tear off your scribbled sheet of paper, or, if you prefer to work in white on a blackboard, visualize yourself wiping away the chalk with a duster. Then, turning the head gently and easily from one shoulder to the other, draw a large infinity sign—a figure of eight, lying on its side. Go over it a dozen times paying attention, as the inward eye travels with the imaginary pencil, to the way in which the successive repetitions of the figure coincide or diverge.

Wipe the blackboard once more, or prepare another clean sheet of paper, and, this time, use your pencil to do a little writing. Begin with your own signature. Because your head and neck move so jerkily, it will look like the signature of an alcoholic illiterate. But practice makes perfect; take a new sheet and begin again. Do this four or five times; then write any other word or phrase that appeals to you.

Like some of the other procedures described above, these drills may seem rather silly, childish and undignified. But this is not important. The important thing is that they work. A little nose-writing, followed by a few minutes of palming, will do wonders in relieving the fatigue of a strained mind and staring eyes, and will result in a perceptible temporary improvement of defective vision. This temporary improvement will become permanent, as the normal and natural functioning fostered by nose-writing and the other procedures described in this book, becomes habitual and automatic.

Mind and body form a single unitary whole. Consequently, such mental processes as remembering and imagining are facilitated by the performance of bodily movements conformable to the objects of our thoughts—the kind of movements we would make if, instead of merely remembering and imagining, we were actually at work upon the things we are thinking about. For example, when remembering or imagining letters or numerals, it is often helpful to place the ball of the thumb in contact with the forefinger and, with it, to print the letters you are working on. Or, alternatively, they may be printed in nose-writing. Or again, if you prefer a more realistic gesture, you may pick up an imaginary pen and trace the signs upon an imaginary notebook.

The aid of the body may also be enlisted through speech. As you remember or imagine a letter, form its name with your lips, or even utter it aloud. The spoken word is so intimately associated with all our processes of thought that any familiar movement of the mouth and vocal cords tends automatically to evoke an image of the thing represented by the articulate sound, which is the product of that movement. Consequently, it is always easier to see what one is reading, when one pronounces the words aloud. People for whom reading is a novelty or a rather difficult and infrequent task—such as children, for example, and the imperfectly educated—realize this fact instinctively. In order to sharpen their vision for the unfamiliar symbols on the page before them, they habitually read aloud. People with defective vision are people, whom their disability has reduced, so to speak, to the cultural ranks. However great their learning, they have become like children or illiterates for whom the printed word is something strange and hard to decipher. This being so, they should, while reacquiring the art of seeing, do the same as the primitives do—form the words they read with their lips and point at them with their fingers. The movement of the organs of speech will evoke auditory and visual images of the words associated with them. Memory and imagination will be stimulated, and the mind will do its work of interpretation, perception and seeing with increased efficiency. Meanwhile the pointing finger (particularly if it is kept almost imperceptibly moving beneath the word which is being looked at) will help to keep the eyes centralized and rapidly shifting over a small area of maximum clarity of vision. In his own way and for his own purposes, the child is eminently wise. When disease or malfunctioning has reduced us, so far as reading is concerned, to the child's level, we should not be ashamed to avail ourselves of this instinctive wisdom.

Chapter 15

Myopia

All persons suffering from defective vision will derive benefit from practicing the fundamental techniques of the art of seeing described in the preceding chapters. In the present chapter and that which follows I shall indicate ways in which certain of these fundamental techniques may be adapted to the needs of persons suffering specifically from nearsightedness, farsightedness, astigmatism and squint, shall also give an account of some new procedures, particularly effective in these various manifestations of disease, hereditary idiosyncrasy and, above all, malfunctioning.

Its Causes

Myopia is almost invariably an acquired condition, which makes its appearance during childhood. It has been attributed to the close work which school children are compelled to perform; and great efforts have been made in all civilized countries to reduce the amount of such work done within a given period, to enlarge the type of textbooks and to improve lighting conditions in schools. The effects of these reforms have been entirely disappointing. Myopia is even commoner today than it was in the past.

This deplorable state of things seems to be due to three principal causes. First, the attempt to improve the environmental conditions prevailing in schools have failed, in certain respects, to go far enough. Second, in other respects, the reforms carried out have been misguided. And third, the reformers have almost completely neglected the psychological reasons for defective vision—a neglect which is particularly serious in the case of children.

It is in the direction of better lighting that the reformers have as yet not gone far enough. Dr. Luckiesh has demonstrated experimentally that visual tasks become easier, and that muscular nervous tension declines, as the intensity of illumination on a given task is increased from one to a hundred foot-candles. He made no experiments with higher intensities, but considers that there is every reason to suppose that muscular nervous tension (the index of strain and fatigue) would continue to fall off with a further increase of illumination to a thousand foot-candles. Now, a child in a well-built, well-lit modern school may think himself extremely lucky if he gets as much as twenty foot-candles of illumination to work with. In many schools he will be given as little as ten or even five. There is reason to believe that many boys and girls might be saved from myopia if they were given sufficient light. In existing conditions only children with the most perfect seeing habits can hope to get through their schooling without straining their organs of vision. But strain is the principal cause of malfunctioning and this, so far as many children are concerned, means myopia.

In their attempt to improve lighting the reformers have not gone far enough. In their attempt to improve the typography of school books they have gone too far in a wrong direction. For the purposes of clear, unstrained seeing, the best print is not necessarily the largest. Large print, it is true, has a specious air of being very easy to read; but precisely because it seems so easy it lures the eyes and mind into temptation. They try to see whole lines of this all too legible print with equal clarity at the same time. Central fixation is lost, the eyes and attention cease to shift, habits of staring are developed and, instead of being improved, vision is actually impaired. For good seeing, the best print is one that is not too large, but fairly heavy, so that there is plenty of strong contrast between the black letters and their background. When confronted by such print the mind and its eyes are not tempted by any obvious excess of legibility to try to see too much too well. Instead, the smaller type encourages them to read with central fixation and in a state of dynamic relaxation. Dr. Bates, indeed, made use of the smallest available print for re-educating defective vision. He would give his pupils not merely diamond type to read (the smallest that a printer can set up), but even those microscopic reductions of print which can only be made by the camera. This microscopic type cannot be read except when the eyes and mind are in a state of complete dynamic relaxation, and are doing their looking with perfect central fixation. With a good teacher to help him a person with even very serious defects of sight (I speak here from personal experience) can be got into the condition in which he can read words printed in microscopic type. And the result is not eyestrain or fatigue, but a marked temporary improvement of vision for other objects. Working with microscopic type without a teacher is not too easy, and the unwary enthusiast may be tempted to set about it in the wrong way. Consequently I have not included any detailed description of this procedure. If I mention it here, it is merely to show that the correlation between large print and good seeing is not the obvious and self-evident thing, which the designers of school books have commonly imagined it to be.

By neglecting the psychological reasons why school children develop defects of vision the reformers have absolutely guaranteed at least a partial failure of their efforts. Even if the lighting of schools were improved out of all recognition, even if the best possible print were used in all of the primers and textbooks, large numbers of children would still undoubtedly develop myopia and other defects of vision. They would do so because they are often bored and sometimes frightened, because they dislike sitting cooped up for long hours, reading and listening to stuff which seems to them largely nonsensical, and compelled to perform tasks which they find not only difficult but pointless. Further, the spirit of competition and the dread of blame or ridicule foster, in many childish minds, a chronic anxiety, which adversely affects every part of the organism, not excluding the eyes and the mental functions associated with seeing. Nor is this all; the exigencies of schooling are such that children must constantly be given novel and unfamiliar things to look at. Every time a new mathematical formula is inscribed on the blackboard, every time the class is set the task of learning a new page of Latin grammar, or to study a new set of features on a map, every child concerned is being forced to pay close and concentrated attention to something completely unfamiliar—that is to say, something which it is peculiarly difficult to see, something which sets up a certain amount of strain in the eyes and minds even of those who have the best of seeing habits.

About seventy percent of children are sufficiently stolid and well balanced to be able to go through school without visual mishap. The rest emerge from the educational ordeal with myopia or some other defect of vision.

Some of the psychological reasons for bad sight can probably never be eliminated from the school; for they seem to be inherent in the very process of herding children together and imposing upon them discipline and book learning. Others can be got rid of—but only by a rare combination of good will and intelligence. (For instance, until all teachers become angels and geniuses, how are you going to prevent a considerable number of children in every generation from being frightened and bored?)

There is, however, one field in which the reasons for bad seeing can be eliminated fairly certainly and without much difficulty: it is possible to mitigate the ocular and mental strain, caused by the constant recurrence of situations in which children are called upon to look at something unfamiliar. The extremely simple technique for achieving this end was devised by Dr. Bates, and for some years was used successfully in a number of schools in different parts of the United States. Owing to changes in the administration of these schools and to pressure exerted by organized orthodoxy, the practices suggested by Dr. Bates were gradually abandoned. The fact is regrettable; for there is evidence that they actually did good in preserving the children's vision, while the nature of the practices was such that it was absolutely impossible that they should ever do anyone any harm.

Dr. Bates' technique for relieving the strain caused by constantly looking at unfamiliar objects was exceedingly simple. It consisted merely in hanging a Snellen chart in some conspicuous position in the school room, and instructing the children, as soon as the chart was thoroughly familiar, to look at it for a few moments whenever they had any difficulty in seeing the blackboard, or a map, or the pages, say, of a grammar or geometry book. Because the chart was an old friend, the children had no difficulty in seeing its graduated letters. The act of reading gave them new faith in their own powers and relieved the strain caused by having to pay concentrated attention to something strange and unfamiliar. Strong in their newfound confidence and relaxation, the children then turned back to their work and found that their power of seeing it had markedly improved.

The Snellen chart possesses, as we have seen, certain disadvantages. Therefore it will probably be advisable to substitute for it a large commercial calendar of the kind described in an earlier chapter. Alternatively, children may be instructed to turn, whenever vision falls off or fatigue sets in, to one of the notices or mottoes which generally hang in school rooms. All that is necessary is that the words, letters or numerals regarded shall be perfectly familiar; for it is by familiarity that the ill effects of unfamiliarity are neutralized.

I need hardly add that there is no reason why this procedure should be confined to the school room. A calendar or any other perfectly memorized piece of printed matter is a valuable addition to the furniture in any room, where people have to do concentrated work involving the seeing of unfamiliar objects, or strange combinations of familiar elements. Incipient strain may be very rapidly relieved by looking—analytically, or with a small-scale swinging shift—at the well-known words or numerals. Add an occasional period of palming and, if possible, of sunning—and there is no reason why the incipient strain should ever mature into fatigue and impairment of vision.

Techniques of Re-education

From this long, but not irrelevant, digression, let us return to a consideration of the procedures for re-educating the myope towards normality. In the more serious cases, the help of a capable teacher will probably be necessary, if any considerable improvement is to be achieved. But all can derive benefit, often a great deal of benefit, from following the fundamental rules of the art of seeing, particularly as these rules are adapted to the special needs of the nearsighted.

Palming, which the myope should practice as often and as long as he possibly can, may be made doubly valuable if the scenes and episodes remembered, while the eyes are closed and covered, are so chosen that the inward eye has to range from near to far over considerable distances. At one time or another, most of us have stood on railway bridges watching the trains as they approached and receded again across the landscape. Such memories are very profitable to the myope; for they stimulate the mind to come out of its narrow world of short sight and plunge into the distance. At the same time, the apparatus of accommodation, which is closely correlated with the mind, is set unconsciously to work.

Friends approaching along familiar roads, horses galloping away across fields, boats gliding along rivers, buses arriving and departing—all such memories of depth and distance are valuable. Sometimes, too, it may be profitable to supplement them with scenes constructed by the fancy. Thus, one may imagine oneself rolling billiard balls down an enormously long table, or flinging a stone onto the ice of a great lake and watching it skim away into the distance.

Sunning and swinging require no special modification for the myope. The drills designed to cure the bad habit of staring and to foster mobility and central fixation can also be performed without modification, except in the case of the calendar drill, which may be adapted to the needs of the nearsighted person in the following ways.

Begin by doing the drills at the distance from which the large numerals can be seen most easily. Do them first with both eyes together, then (covering one eye with a patch or handkerchief) with each eye separately. If one eye does its work of sensing less well than the other, give it more work—but lengthen the periods of palming between drills, so as to avoid fatigue. After a few days when the eyes and mind have become accustomed to doing a certain amount of seeing without the aid of spectacles (which will still have to be worn in times of emergency, or of potential danger to oneself or others, as when driving a car or walking in crowded streets), move the chair a foot or two further from the calendar and repeat the drills at that distance. In a few weeks it should be possible to increase very considerably the distance from which things can be clearly seen.

Myopic eyes should be given plenty of practice in changing the focus from the near point to the distance. To do this, procure a small pocket calendar of the same model as the commercial calendar on the wall—that is to say, with one month printed in large type, and the preceding and succeeding months in smaller type below. Hold the pocket calendar a few inches in front of the eyes, glance at the figure "one" on the large-type month, then look away and locate the "one" on the large-type month of the wall calendar. Close the eyes and relax. Then proceed to do the same with the succeeding figures. All the steps of the drill may be done in this way on the two calendars, with both eyes together and each eye separately and at progressively greater and greater distances from the wall calendar. Nearsighted people will find this a pretty strenuous exercise, and should therefore be particularly careful to interrupt the drill at frequent intervals for periods of palming and, if possible, sunning. If a small pocket calendar does not happen, on some occasion, to be available, the face of a watch may be used instead. Hold it close to the eyes, glance at the "one" and then away to the corresponding numeral on the wall calendar. Close the eyes, relax and go on in the same way round the whole dial.

Myopes can read without glasses, but at a point abnormally close to the eyes. It is possible for them, however, to read without undue strain at points an inch or two further away. Practice in reading at these further points will gradually eliminate any slight feeling of discomfort associated with the more distant vision—provided always, of course, that attention be properly directed and staring (the great vice of the nearsighted) avoided. At the end of every page, or even of every paragraph, the myope should look up for a few seconds to glance at some thoroughly familiar object at a distance, such as a calendar on the wall, or the view out of the window. Further hints on the art of reading will be given in the chapter especially devoted to that subject.

When travelling by bus or car, myopes should take the opportunity provided of glancing with quick, "flashing" regards at the lettering on billboards, shop fronts and the like. No attempt should be made to "hold" the words so regarded, until they are clearly seen. Glance for a moment, and close the eyes. Then, if the movement of the vehicle permits it, glance again. If you see, well and good; if you don't see, that also is well and good—for there is every reason to believe that you will see better some time.

A few hints on the art of seeing movies will be given in a later chapter. Here I will only remark that for anyone who can bear to look at a picture more than once, the movie theatre may be made to provide material for a valuable exercise. On your first visit, look at the picture from a place in one of the front rows. On the next, take a seat twenty feet further back. Because of its familiarity the picture will be more visible than it was the first time; and you will see it well even at the increased distance. Yet greater familiarity will, on a third visit, permit of a further retreat towards the back of the theatre. And, of course, if your courage, time and money are sufficient, you can view the picture for a fourth, a fifth, a sixth, a seventy times seventh time, creeping further and further away from the screen on each occasion.

Chapter 16

Long Sight, Astigmatism, Squint

Long sight, or farsightedness, is of two main types—hyperopia, often found in young people and persisting into later life; and presbyopia, which commonly makes its onset in later middle age. All forms of farsightedness can be re-educated into or towards normality.

Hyperopia often causes discomfort and pain, and when associated (as it not infrequently is) with a very slight degree of outward squint in one of the eyes, may bring on frequent severe headaches, giddiness, fits of nausea and vomiting. The neutralizing of hyperopic symptoms by means of artificial lenses sometimes puts a stop to these painful disabilities; but sometimes it fails to do so, and the migraines and nausea persist until such time as the sufferer learns the art of seeing.

Presbyopia is commonly regarded as one of the inevitable results of aging. Like the bones of the skeleton, the lens of the eye hardens with age, and this hardening is supposed to prevent all elderly eyes from being able to accommodate at the near point. Nevertheless, many old people continue to accommodate up to the day of their death; and when sufferers from presbyopia undertake a suitable course of visual re-education, they soon learn to read at a normal distance without the aid of spectacles. From this we may conclude that there is nothing inevitable or predestined about the farsightedness of old age.

Palming, sunning, swinging and shifting will do much to relieve the discomfort associated with hyperopia, and will put the mind and eyes into the condition of dynamic relaxation which makes normal seeing possible. These should be supplemented by imagination drills, which are particularly valuable in improving the farsighted person's ability to read.

Print seems grey and blurred when the hyperope looks at it. This state of things can be improved indirectly by a constant practice of the fundamental procedures of the art of seeing—palming, sunning, swinging and shifting; and, directly, through memory and imagination. The hyperope should look at one of the large numerals on his calendar and then, with closed eyes, "letting go" remember the intense blackness of the ink and reflect at the same time that exactly the same ink is used for printing the small letters, which he sees as grey and misty. Next, calling imagination into play, he should remember one of these smaller letters, imagine a blacker dot at its base and another at the top. After shifting from dot to dot with the inward eye, he should look at the real letter and do the same with that. It will soon blacken and, for a few seconds, he will be able to see it and the other letters on the page quite distinctly. Then all will blur again, and he will have to repeat his acts of memory and imagination.

After paying attention for a little to the blackness of the letters, he should consider the whiteness of the background within and around the letters, and should exercise himself in first imagining and then, with the aid of the imagination, actually seeing it whiter than it is in reality. The vision for reading and other close work may be markedly improved in this way. This is not surprising; for between the eyes and the mind there exists a two-way connection. A mental strain will cause strain and physical distortion in the eyes; and physical distortion in the eyes will cause the mind to perceive an imperfect image of the external object, and so increase its strain. But, conversely, if the mind is able, through memory and imagination, to form within itself a perfect image of an external object, the existence of this perfect image in the mind will automatically improve the condition of the strained and distorted eyes. The more perfect the image in the mind, the greater the improvement in the physical condition of the eyes. For the eyes will tend to assume the physical conformation, which eyes must have, if they are to transmit the sort of *sensa* that a mind can perceive in terms of a perfect image of an external object. Not only is the connection between eyes and mind a reversible, two-way connection; it is also a connection for mutual benefit as well as for mutual harm. This is a very important fact to remember; for we tend, for some curious reason, to think only of the mischief that the eyes can inflict upon the mind and the mind upon the eyes—of blurred vision, due to strain and refractive error, and of visual delusions produced by the imagination, of temporary failures of vision caused by sudden outbursts of rage or grief, and of diseases of the eyes brought on by chronic negative emotion. But if eyes and mind can harm, they can also help one another. An unstrained mind has undistorted eyes, and undistorted eyes do their work so well that they never add anything to the burdens of the mind. Moreover, when, through mental strain or for some other reason, a distortion of the eyes has been produced, the mind can help to remedy this distortion by doing the right, the beneficial thing at its end of the two-way communication line. It can perform acts of remembering, which are always accompanied by the condition of relaxation that permits the eyes to return to their normal shape and normal functioning. And it can call up, by imagination, representations of external objects more perfect than those it ordinarily sees on the basis of the poor *sensa* transmitted by the distorted eyes. But when the mind has a perfectly clear image of an object, the eyes tend automatically to revert to the condition which would enable them to furnish the proper raw materials for making such an image. Just as the emotions and their outward physical expression (in the form of gesture, metabolic change, glandular activity and so forth) are indissolubly connected, so too there is an indissoluble connection, for good as well as for evil, between the visual image, whether produced by memory, imagination or the interpretation of *sensa*, and the physical condition of the eyes. Impair or improve the mental image, and you automatically impair or improve the condition of the eyes. By means of repeated acts of memory and imagination it is possible to improve, temporarily at first, then permanently, the quality of the mental images of external objects. When this has been achieved there is first a temporary, then a permanent improvement in the physical condition of the eyes. Hence the value of memory and imagination drills in conditions such as hyperopia, in which *sensa* and the perceptions based upon them are of poor quality.

Exercises which compel the mind and eyes to change their focus rapidly from distance to the near point are as useful to the hyperope as to the myope. Such drills have already been described in the chapter on short sight.

Presbyopia is essentially an inability to accommodate the eyes, so that they will do clear and accurate sensing at the near point. This failure to accommodate seems to be the result of a habit, to the building up of which middle-aged and elderly people are predisposed by the hardening of the lens. This habit can, as experience shows, be modified, even though the physical condition of the lens may remain, as it presumably does, unchanged. Like all other sufferers from defects of vision, presbyopes should follow the fundamental rules of the art of seeing, adapting them to their own particular needs and, where necessary, supplementing them. To the procedures which are helpful to all farsighted persons, they should add the following techniques for improving their reading.

Print can be read without undue strain somewhat nearer to the eyes than the point of maximum comfort and habitual usage. The presbyope can coax his eyes and mind to get used to seeing at this nearer point, provided always that he interrupts his reading to keep the visual organs relaxed by means of palming, swinging and sunning. Little by little, the reading distance can be considerably shortened in this way, while the eyes and mind acquire a renewal of flexibility.

Oliver Wendell Holmes records the case of an old gentleman of his acquaintance who, "perceiving his sight to fail, immediately took to exercising it on the finest print, and in this way fairly bullied nature out of her foolish habit of taking liberties at five-and-forty, or thereabout. And now the old gentleman performs the most extraordinary feats with his pen, showing that his eyes must be a pair of microscopes. I should be afraid to say how much he writes on the compass of a half-dime—whether the Psalms or the Gospels, or the Psalms and the Gospels, I won't be positive."

This old gentleman had evidently discovered for himself what Dr. Bates was later to rediscover and proclaim to the world—the value, for people with defective sight, of very small and even microscopic print. Oliver Wendell Holmes is wrong, however, in saying that he "fairly bullies nature out of her habit" of giving people presbyopia. The sensing eyes and the perceiving mind cannot successfully be bullied. Any attempt to force them to sense and perceive always results, within a very short time, not in the improvement of vision, but its impairment. The old gentleman who trained his eyes to become a pair of microscopes cannot possibly have bullied; he must have coaxed them. And provided they do the same, all presbyopes may profitably follow his example.

Procure a specimen of very small print. (In any second-hand bookshop you may find thick little duodecimos of the early nineteenth century, containing the complete works of the great and the forgotten, and printed in a diamond type so small that our ancestors must indeed have had good vision to get through whole volumes of it.) Take the sunlight on the closed eyes, or, if there is no sun, bathe them in the light of a strong electric lamp. Palm for a few minutes, and then give the closed eyes a few more seconds of light. Thus relaxed, you can set to work on your small print. Holding the page either in full sunlight, or in the best possible substitute for sunlight, look at it easily, effortlessly, breathing and blinking as you do so. Make no attempt to see the words, but let the eyes wander back and forth along the white spaces between the lines of print. No mental hazards are involved in looking at a plain surface; consequently, there will be no temptation to strain if you keep the eyes and attention shifting on the white spaces between the lines. From far out, move the page to within a foot of the eyes, still paying attention to the white spaces rather than the print, and still taking care to breathe and blink, so as to prevent the attention from becoming unduly fixed and immobile. (By changing the outward expression of an undesirable mental state, one acts upon the mental state itself. Attention cannot be misdirected, if we take pains to correct the external symptoms of misdirected attention.) Interrupt this procedure at frequent intervals to palm and take the sun. This is essential; for, as we have seen, there can be no bullying of the sensing eyes and the perceiving mind. If they are to cooperate in doing a good job of seeing, they must be relaxed and coaxed into working as they should.

After a little time devoted to this drill, it will generally be found that individual words and whole phrases of the small-type reading matter will come up almost suddenly into distinct visibility. Do not allow yourself to be tempted by these first successes into trying to read continuously. Your aim at this time is not to reach the immediate and obvious goal of reading the page before you; it is to acquire the means whereby this and similar goals may be reached in the future, without strain or fatigue, and with enhanced efficiency. Do not, I repeat, attempt to read, but go on effortlessly regarding the page, and especially the white spaces between the lines, at varying distances from the eyes. From time to time, when a word in the small type has come up into visibility, pick up a book with print of ordinary dimensions and read a paragraph or two. It is quite likely that you will find you can read it more easily and closer to the eyes than you could before starting your work on the smaller print.

Astigmatism and Squint

Defects of vision, due to astigmatism, can be markedly diminished or even eliminated by anyone who will diligently practice the art of seeing and thereby learn how to get his mind and eyes to function naturally and normally. Procedures especially valuable for the astigmatic have already been described in the paragraphs devoted to the domino drills. It is therefore unnecessary to go any further into the matter here.

Sufferers from any of the more serious kinds of squint will find it extremely difficult to re-educate themselves into normality, and should seek the assistance of an experienced teacher, who will show them how to achieve dynamic relaxation, how to strengthen the sight of the weaker eye, and (final and most difficult step) how to reacquire the mental faculty of fusing the two sets of *sensa* delivered by the two eyes into a single representation of an external object.

For those who suffer from slight muscle imbalance—and even an almost imperceptible divergence of one or both eyes may be the source of extreme discomfort and often of serious disabilities—the following simple "double-image drill" will prove of considerable benefit.

Relax the eyes and mind by palming; then hold a pencil at arms length, the tip pointed towards your nose. Bring the pencil towards you, blinking as you do so. When the pencil is close to the face, change its position from horizontal to vertical, holding it upright immediately in front of, and about three inches away from, the tip of the nose. Focus on the pencil; but, to avoid staring, shift the attention rapidly from top to bottom. Do this half a dozen times; then look away, just above the the top of the pencil, to some distant object at the other end of the room. When the eyes are focused on this distant object the pencil at the near point will seem to become two pencils. To eyes in perfect alignment, these two pencils will look as though they were about three inches apart. But where there is muscular imbalance, the distance separating the two images will appear to be a good deal less. (And if the squint is pronounced, the phenomenon will not be observed at all.) Should the two images be seen too close together, shut the eyes, "let go" and imagine yourself still looking at the distant object, but with the two images of the nearby pencil somewhat further apart than they were when you actually saw them. When we distinctly imagine a normal image, our eyes will tend automatically to put themselves into the condition in which they would have to be in order to supply our mind with the materials for seeing such an image. Consequently, when you reopen the eyes and look once more in reality at the distant object, the two pencils at the near point will seem, if your visualization has been clear and distinct, perceptibly further apart than they were. Close the eyes again and repeat the visualizing process, this time imagining the pencils to be yet a little further apart than before; then reopen and verify. Go on doing this until you have pushed the two images to something like their normal distance one from the other. When this has been achieved, start to swing the head very gently from side to side, blinking and breathing easily as you do so—and, of course, still looking at the distant object. The two images of the pencil will appear to move back and forth in the opposite direction to the head, but will still keep their positions relative to one another.

Provided that this drill be prepared for by palming and accompanied by easy blinking and breathing, it may be repeated at frequent intervals throughout the day. The immediate result will be, not fatigue, but relaxation and de-tensioning; and the long-range consequences will be the gradual correction of old established habits of muscular imbalance.

Diseases of the Eyes

The art of seeing is not primarily a therapy. It does not, that is to say, aim directly at the cure of pathological conditions of the sensing apparatus. Its purpose is to promote normal and natural functioning of the organs of vision—the sensing eyes and the selecting, perceiving and seeing mind. When normal and natural functioning has been restored, it generally happens that there is a marked improvement in the organic condition of the tissues involved in that functioning.

In this particular case, the tissues involved are those of the eyes and the nerves and muscles connected with them. When people have learned the art of seeing and conscientiously follow its simple rules, their eyes, if these are diseased, tend to get better. Even when the disease has its origin in some other part of the body, normal and natural visual functioning will often bring a certain amelioration in the local condition of the eyes. It cannot, of course, eliminate the condition altogether, for the simple reason that the sickness of the eyes is only a symptom of another sickness having its seat elsewhere. It can, however, help the eyes while the cause of their disorder is being treated, and may do much to prevent the vision from suffering permanent impairment.

In cases where the pathological condition of the eyes is not a symptom of a disease in some other part of the body, the re-establishment of normal and natural functioning may lead indirectly to a complete cure. This, as I have said before, is only to be expected; for habitual malfunctioning results in chronic nervous muscular tension and reduction in the volume of circulation. But any part of the body in which circulation is inadequate is particularly susceptible to disease; furthermore, once disease has set in, the innate capacity of the organ to regulate and heal itself will be abnormally reduced. Any procedure which restores normal functioning to the psycho-physical organs of vision will tend to reduce nervous muscular tension, increase circulation and bring back the *vis medicatrix naturae* to its normal potency. Experience shows that this is what in effect generally occurs when persons suffering from such conditions as glaucoma, cataract, iritis and detachment of the retina learn how to use their eyes and minds properly instead of improperly. The art of seeing, I repeat, is not primarily a therapy; but, at one remove and indirectly, it results in the relief or cure of many serious diseases of the eyes.

Chapter 17

Some Difficult Seeing Situations

In the present chapter I propose to discuss the ways in which the fundamental rules of the art of seeing may be applied to certain common situations which persons with defective vision are apt to find particularly trying.

Reading

When we read we are assailed, if our vision is at all defective, by particularly strong temptations to use our eyes and mind in the wrong way. Our interest in what we read intensifies our all too human proclivity towards end-gaining. We are so greedy to see the greatest possible amount of print in the shortest possible time, that we utterly neglect the normal and natural means whereby such an end may be achieved. Improper functioning becomes habitual with us, and our vision is further impaired.

The first thing we have to do is to realize that end-gaining is self-stultifying, and that where reading is concerned we ourselves are end-gainers. The next is to inhibit, whenever we read, the manifestations of our impatience and our intellectual gluttony.

In the early stages of visual re-education clear and effortless reading cannot be accomplished without plenty of rest and relaxation. In other words, relaxation is one of the principal means whereby we can achieve our end, which is to see as much print as possible in the shortest possible time, with the least possible fatigue and the highest degree of intellectual efficiency. Consequently, when we inhibit the manifestations of our impatience and greed, this should be done, first of all, for the sake of giving our eyes and minds the relaxation which they so urgently need, but of which they are perpetually depriving themselves through their habits of improper use.

To provide the eyes and mind with adequate relaxation, one should, while reading, adopt the following simple procedures.

First: Close the eyes for a second or two at the end of every sentence, or every other sentence. "Let go" and visualize the last word you have read and the punctuation mark by which it is followed. When you open your eyes again, look first at this remembered word and punctuation mark, which will seem to be perceptibly more distinct than they were when originally read. Then go on to the next sentence.

Second: At the end of every page or two, interrupt yourself for a couple of minutes to palm the eyes. To greedy end-gainers, this will seem the most intolerable hardship. But let them reflect that these interruptions will bring them more easily and expeditiously to their goal. Also that this "mortification" of their impatience will probably be very good for their characters!

Third: If sunlight is available, take the sun on the closed and open eyes before palming, and again, on the closed lids, after. If there is no sun, bathe the eyes in the light of a strong electric lamp.

Fourth: While reading, sit where you can see a calendar or other perfectly familiar piece of large-type reading matter hanging on a distant wall. Raise your eyes from your book occasionally and look analytically at the letters or numerals. If you are reading by daylight, look out of the window sometimes into the far distance.

Fifth: Memory and imagination can be enlisted in the service of better reading. Pause from time to time, "let go" and remember a single letter or word recently regarded. See it with the inward eye in terms of the white background surrounding it and contained within it. Then imagine the whiteness of the background as being whiter than you actually saw it. Reopen, look at the whiteness around and within the real letters, and try to see it as white as the imaginary background you visualized with your eyes shut. Close the eyes once more, and begin again. After two or three repetitions, palm for a little while and then go on reading.

As an alternative exercise, close your eyes, remember a recently seen letter, take an imaginary pen and place a dot of intenser blackness at its top and base, or at its left hand and right hand extremities. Shift the attention from dot to dot half a dozen times; then open the eyes and, imagining that you see similar dots of intenser blackness of the real letter, do the same. Repeat this procedure several times, palm and continue your reading.

Sixth: In the chapter on farsightedness, I gave an account of the way in which presbyopes could improve their reading vision by looking effortlessly at very small print—more especially at the white spaces between the lines. The benefits of this drill are not confined to elderly people with failing sight. Anyone who has difficulty in reading may profitably make use of this procedure at the beginning of a period of study, and at intervals during the period.

So much for the simple relaxation techniques, by which a session with book or newspaper should be prefaced and interrupted. Let us now consider the proper way of performing the act of reading itself.

Here, as in all other seeing situations, the great enemies of normal vision are strain, misdirected attention, staring. In order to overcome these enemies, one must be careful, while reading, to obey the following simple rules.

First: Do not hold your breath or keep the eyelids rigid and unmoving for long periods. Blink frequently and breathe regularly, gently and fully.

Second: Do not stare or try to see every part of a whole line or phrase equally well. Keep the eyes and attention continually moving, and so bring central fixation into play. This is best accomplished by making the eyes hurry continuously back and forth in the white space immediately under the line of print which is being read. Words and letters are thus caught, as it were, between a succession of short swings. At first this technique of reading by rapid movements of the eyes in the white spaces between the lines may seem somewhat disconcerting. But after a little time we shall discover that it contributes not a little to clear and effortless reading. Letters and words are seen more easily when they are, so to speak, on the wing than when immobilized by a fixed stare—more easily, too, when they are considered as interruptions to a plain white background than when looked at as things existing in their own right and requiring to be deciphered.

Third: do not frown when you read. Frowning is a symptom of the nervous muscular tension produced in and around the eyes by misdirected attention and the effort to see. With the achievement of dynamic relaxation and normal functioning, the habit of frowning will disappear of itself. But its departure may be accelerated, and the physical and mental tensions relieved, by frequent and deliberate acts of inhibition. In the midst of reading, suddenly turn round upon yourself and catch your facial muscles at their tricks. Then close the eyes for a moment, "let go" and deliberately smooth the brows.

Fourth: Do not half-close the eyelids when you read. Unlike frowning, this procedure has a purpose. By half-closing the eyelids, we reduce the size of the normal visual field and, in this way, eliminate some of the distracting stimuli and diffused illumination coming to the eyes from those parts of the page which are not being looked at. Most persons with defects of vision do their reading through a narrow loophole between their eyelashes; but the tendency is especially marked among those who have opacities in the cornea or other normally transparent tissues of the eyes. Such opacities act in much the same way as do the particles of water vapor suspended in the air on an autumn morning: they disperse the light in a kind of luminous fog, through which it is hard to see distinctly. Partial closure of the lids has the effect of cutting off much of the illuminated field and so reducing the density of the fog caused by the scattering of light.

But the narrowing of the aperture between the lids demands a continuous muscular effort. This effort increases the tension in and around the eyes, and is reflected by an intensification of the psychological tensions in the mind. Looking between half-closed lids is undoubtedly a way of getting an immediate improvement of vision; but this immediate improvement must be paid for in the future—for it can be had only at the high cost of increased strain and fatigue, and a progressive further impairment of the power of seeing. It is therefore very important to find a method for correcting this most undesirable tendency. Conscious relaxation of the lids, so that they remain untensed and open at their normal span, will not be sufficient. Indeed, it is likely to result in our seeing a good deal worse than before, so that, in mere self-protection, we shall have to turn back to our old bad habits.

Fortunately, however, there is a very simple mechanical method for getting the results achieved by half-closing the eyes. Instead of cutting out distractions and unneeded illumination at the receiving end, that is to say, in the eye, we cut them out at the source—on the printed page. All that is needed is a sheet of stout black paper, a ruler and a sharp knife. Take as much of the black paper as will cover, say, half an average page of print. Across the center of this cut a slot slightly longer than the average line of print and wide enough to take in about two lines. (The width of the slot may be varied to suit individual tastes and to fit different sizes of type. This can be done by taking a strip of black paper, drawing it down across the top edge of the slot until the aperture is of the width desired, and fastening it into place by paper clips.)

When everything is ready, hold the black paper flat on the page with the lower edge of the slot about an eighth of an inch below the line you are reading. When you have come to the end of the line, move the slot down to the next line. And so on.

This absurdly simple little device will be found helpful by all who have any difficulty in reading. For those who suffer from corneal or other opacities, it may double the clarity of their reading vision— and this when the eyelids are fully open and relaxed.

Reading through a slot facilitates that anti-stare technique of which I have already spoken—the rapid shifting to and fro on the white space immediately under the print. The straight edge of the black paper acts as a sort of railway track, along which the eyes travel easily and smoothly. Furthermore, the task of imaginatively seeing the white spaces between lines as whiter than they really are is facilitated when these white spaces are regarded (and afterwards remembered) in contact with a contrasting black frame.

In certain cases the habit of trying to see clearly too much print at the same time may be rapidly corrected by making use of a small slot, not more than three quarters of an inch long. Such a slot will permit its user to see only so much of any given line as can be taken in by the *macula lutea*; and rapid shifting within this confined space will bring the *fovea* into play. In this way the central area of the retina will be stimulated and set to work as it never was when the impossible attempt was made to see whole phrases and lines equally well at the same time. The short slot will have to be moved rapidly from word to word along the line, and reading with its aid will probably be found rather exasperating, at any rate in the beginning. To minimize this inconvenience, alternate between the long slot and the short. It is easy to put up with brief annoyances, particularly if one reflects that by doing so one is building up profitable habits of corneal visual functioning.

Looking at Unfamiliar Objects

This is perhaps the most trying of all seeing situations and also one of frequent occurrence. We are called upon to look intensively at unfamiliar objects every time we go shopping, visit a museum, search for books in the shelves of a library, hunt through drawers and cupboards for some lost article, tidy up attic, pack and unpack baggage, or repair a machine. The problem is how to avoid or reduce the strain and fatigue that ordinarily follows such looking.

First of all, make sure, if this is in your power, that what you are looking at is brightly illuminated. Draw back curtains, turn on lights, use a flashlight. However, if the looking has to be done in some public place, you will have to put up with the lighting which others consider sufficient but which will almost certainly be inadequate.

Second, resist the temptation to stare, and do not try to see clearly more than a small part of the total visual field. Look analytically at what is before you, and keep the eyes and attention continuously shifting.

Third, do not hold your breath, and blink your eyes frequently.

Fourth, rest as often as you can, either closing the eyes, "letting go" and remembering some familiar object, or, preferably, palming. If possible sun the eyes from time to time, or bathe them in the light of an electric lamp.

If these simple rules are followed, it should be possible to come through the ordeal without serious fatigue, discomfort or strain.

Movies

For many people with defective vision a visit to the movies may be the cause of much fatigue and discomfort. There is no need for this. Looked at in the right way, movies do not strain the eyes and, indeed, may be made to pay handsome dividends in improved vision. Here are the rules which must be followed, if an evening at the picture theatre is to be a pleasure not a torture.

First: Refrain from staring. Do not try to see the whole of the screen equally well. Do not try to "hold" any detail. On the contrary, keep the eyes and attention continuously on the move.

Second: Do not forget to breathe and blink regularly.

Third: Take the opportunity offered by boring sequences to rest, by closing the eyes for a few seconds and "letting go." Even during the more exciting parts of the picture, you can find time occasionally to glance away for an instant into the darkness surrounding the illuminated screen. Use any intermission for palming.

One way in which the movies may be used for improving vision has already been described in the chapter on myopia. Movies are also helpful in other ways, above all by making it possible for us to become familiar with objects and situations which are frequently met with in real life.

In an essay on the relationship between life and art, Roger Fry has written a passage which casts a very interesting light on the way in which the movies can be used to improve defective vision. "We can get a curious side glimpse," he writes in *Vision and Design*, "of the nature of the imaginative life from the cinematograph. This resembles actual life in almost every respect, except that what the psychologists call the conative part of our reaction to sensations, that is to say, the appropriate resultant action, is cut off. If, in a cinematograph, we see a runaway horse and cart, we do not have to think of getting out of the way, or heroically interposing ourselves. The result is that, in the first place, we *see*. the event much more clearly; see a number of quite interesting but irrelevant things, which in real life could not struggle into our consciousness, bent, as it would be, entirely upon the problems of our appropriate reaction. I remember seeing in a cinematograph the arrival of a train at a foreign station, and the people descending from the carriages; there was no platform, and to my intense surprise, I saw several people turn right around, after reaching the ground, as though to orientate themselves; an almost ridiculous performance, which I had never noticed in all the many hundred occasions on which such a scene had passed before my eyes in real life. The fact being that, at a station, one is never really a spectator of events, but an actor engaged in the drama of luggage or prospective seats; and one actually sees only so much as may help to the appropriate action."

These lines express a very important truth: there is a fundamental psychological difference between a spectator and an actor, between looking on at a work of art and looking on (which can rarely be done without intervening) at an episode of real life. Spectators see more, and more clearly, than do actors. Owing to this fact, it is possible to make use of the movies to improve our vision for objects and events in real life. Because you are not a participant in the drama, you will be able to see more clearly than you could in real life the way in which people on the screen perform such ordinary acts as opening a door, getting into a cab, helping themselves to food and so forth. Make yourself conscious of seeing more on the screen than you are normally able to do in real life, and after the show deliberately call back the memory-images of what you saw there. This will make such ordinary actions seem more familiar than before; and this increased familarity will cause similar actions to be more visible to you when they occur at some future date in real life.

Close-ups provide a means whereby persons with defective vision may overcome one of their most embarrassing handicaps— the inability to recognize faces, or to catch the fine shades of meaning which people normally convey through facial expression. In real life faces sixteen feet high and eight feet wide are unknown; but on the screen they are one of the most ordinary of phenomena. Exploit this fact in such a way as to improve your vision for real faces of ordinary dimensions. Look carefully at the gigantic face. Carefully, but always analytically. Never fix a greedy stare upon a closeup, even if it should belong to your favorite star. Examine it in all its details, noting the structure of the bones, the way the hair grows, and how the head moves on the neck and the eyes within their orbits. And when the colossal face registers grief, desire, anger, doubt and the rest, follow the workings of lips and eyes, of the muscles of cheek and brow, with the closest attention. The more carefully and analytically you observe these things, the better and clearer will be your memories of the commoner facial expressions, and the easier will it be at some later date to see similar expressions on the faces of real people.

Chapter 18

Lighting Conditions

People with normal vision who consistently do their sensing and perceiving in a condition of dynamic relaxation can afford in large measure to disregard the external conditions of seeing. Not so the men and women whose sight is defective. For them favorable external conditions are of the greatest importance, and the failure to secure such favorable conditions may do much to increase their disability, or, if they have undertaken a course of visual re-education, to retard their progress towards normality.

The most important all the external conditions of good seeing is adequate illumination. Where lighting is poor it is very hard for people with defective vision to get better, very easy for them to get worse.

The question now arises, what *is* adequate illumination?

The best illumination we have is full sunshine on a clear summer's day. If you read in such sunshine, the intensity of the light falling upon the page of your book will be in the neighborhood of ten thousand foot-candles—that is to say, the light of direct summer sunshine is equal to the light thrown by ten thousand wax candles placed at the distance of one foot from the book. Move from full sunlight to the shade of a tree or a house. The light on your page will still have an intensity of about one thousand foot-candles. On overcast days the light reflected from white clouds has an intensity of several thousand foot-candles; and the weather must be very gloomy for general outdoor intensities to fall as low as a thousand foot-candles.

Indoors, the light near an unobstructed window may have an intensity of anything from one hundred to five hundred foot-candles, depending upon the brightness of the day. Ten or fifteen feet away from the window the illumination may fall to as little as two foot-candles or even less, if the room is papered and furnished in dark colors.

The intensity of illumination diminishes as the square of the distance. A sixty-watt lamp will provide about eighty foot-candles at one foot, about twenty at two feet, about nine at three feet, and, at ten feet, only four-fifths of one foot-candle. Owing to this rapid falling off in intensity with increase of distance, most parts of the average artificially lighted room are very poorly illuminated. It is common to find people reading and doing other forms of close work under an illumination of one or two foot-candles. In public buildings such as schools and libraries you will be lucky if you get as much as five foot-candles of illumination.

That it should be possible to do close work under illuminations so fantastically low compared with those which are met with out-of-doors in daytime is a remarkable tribute to the native endurance and flexibility of the sensing eyes and the perceiving mind. So great is this flexibility and endurance that a person whose eyes are unimpaired, and who uses them in the way that nature intended them to be used, can submit for long periods to bad lighting conditions and suffer no harm. But for a person whose eyes have undergone some organic impairment, or whose habitual functioning is so unnatural that he can only see with effort and under strain, these same conditions may be disastrous.

In his book, *Seeing and Human Welfare*, Dr. Luckiesh has described some very interesting experiments which demonstrate the undesirable consequences of poor lighting. These experiments were designed to measure nervous muscular tension (an accurate indicator, as Dr. Luckiesh points out, of "strain, fatigue, wasted effort and internal losses") under varying conditions of illumination. The task assigned to the subjects of these experiments was reading; and the amount of nervous muscular strain was recorded by a device which measured the pressure exerted by two fingers of the left hand resting upon a large flat knob. The subjects were kept unaware of the nature and purpose of the investigation—indeed, were deliberately thrown on a wrong scent. This eliminated the possibility of any conscious or voluntary interference with the results. A very large number of tests showed conclusively that in all cases "there was a large decrease in nervous muscular tension as the intensity increased from one to one hundred foot-candles. The latter was the highest intensity investigated, because this is far above prevailing levels of illumination in the artificial world. There was impressive evidence that this tension would continue to decrease if the level of illumination were increased to 1000 foot-candles." In other tests the subjects were exposed to improperly placed lights that threw a glare in their eyes. This glare was not excessive—just the average, moderate glare that millions of human beings habitually work and play by. Nevertheless it was quite sufficient to increase the telltale nervous muscular tension to a marked degree.

There is, so far as I know, only one kind of electric light bulb from which one can obtain a thousand foot-candles of illumination without excessive consumption of current. That is the 150-watt spotlight, described in the chapter on sunning. The parabolic and silvered back of this bulb acts as a reflector, and the light issues in a powerful beam, in which reading, sewing and other tasks requiring close attention and precise seeing can be performed in the best possible conditions.

During the daytime people with defective sight should always make use of the best illumination available. Whenever possible close work should be done near a window or out of doors. I myself have derived great benefit from reading for long periods at a stretch in full sunlight, either falling directly on the page, or, if the weather was too hot, reflected by means of an adjustable mirror, so that it was possible to sit in the shade, or indoors, and to enjoy the advantage of seven or eight thousand foot-candles upon the book. For some months, indeed, after giving up the wearing of spectacles, it was only in full sunlight, or under a spot lamp, that I could read comfortably for any length of time. But as vision improved, it became possible for me to make use of less intense illuminations. I still, however, prefer the spotlight to all others, and frequently work in full sunlight.

When reading in full sunlight, it is necessary to keep the eyes thoroughly relaxed by means of periodical brief sunnings and palmings. Many people will also find it easier to read if they make use of a slot cut in black paper, as described in an earlier chapter. When these precautions are taken, reading under ten thousand foot-candles can be very helpful to those whose vision is defective. Falling upon the center of sight, the image of the intensely illuminated print stimulates a *macula* which has become sluggish and insensitive through habitual wrong use of the organs of seeing. At the same time, the clarity and distinctness of the sunlit letters exercise a most wholesome influence upon the mind, which loses its habitual strained anxiety about seeing and acquires instead an easy confidence in its ability to interpret the *sensa* brought to it by the eyes. Thanks to this confidence and to the stimulation of the sluggish *macula*, it becomes possible, after a time, to do one's seeing no less effectively under lower intensities of illumination. Ten thousand foot-candles reading is a preparation and an education for hundred foot-candle reading.

Owing sometimes to organic defects of the eyes, sometimes to ingrained habits of improper functioning, sometimes to generalized ill-health, certain persons are peculiarly sensitive to intense light. For these it would be unwise to plunge directly into ten thousand foot-candle reading. Following the techniques described in the chapter on sunning, they should gradually accustom themselves to tolerate greater and greater intensities of illumination, not only directly on the closed and open eyes, but also on the printed page before them. In this way, they will come by slow degrees to be able to enjoy the advantages of good lighting—advantages from which their organic or functional photophobia had previously cut them off, forcing them to strain for vision in a perpetual twilight.

In conclusion, it seems worthwhile to say a few words about the fluorescent lighting, now so extensively used in factories, shops and offices, on account of its cheapness. There is good evidence that this kind of lighting adversely affects the vision of a minority of those who have to do close work under it. One reason for this must be sought in the composition of the light itself, which does not come from an incandescent source, as does natural sunlight or the light from a filament bulb. Nor is this all. Fluorescent lighting throws almost no shadows. Consequently the element of contrast, so immensely important to normal seeing, is conspicuously absent from rooms illuminated by fluorescent tubes. Shadows, moreover, help us in our estimation of distances, forms and textures. When shadows are absent, we are deprived of one of our most valuable guideposts to reality, and the accurate interpretation of *sensa* becomes much harder. This is one of the reasons why the organs of vision tire so much more easily on a day of uniform high cloud than on one of bright sunshine. Fluorescent lighting produces an effect somewhat similar to that produced by the diffused glare reflected from high thin clouds. To eyes that have been evolved to adapt themselves to light proceeding from an incandescent source, and to minds that have learned to make use of shadows as guides to correct interpretation, perception and judgment, fluorescent lighting cannot but seem strange and baffling. The wonder is that it is only a minority of people who react unfavorably to such lighting.

If you happen to belong to the unlucky ten or fifteen percent of the population which cannot work under fluorescent light without suffering from bloodshot eyes, swollen eyelids and lowered vision, the best thing you can do, of course, is to find a job which permits you to work out-of-doors, or by the light of incandescent filament lamps. The next best thing is to palm frequently, and get out of the fluorescence as often as possible for a few minutes of sunning. At night, as a substitute for sunning, take the light of a strong incandescent filament lamp upon the closed and open eyes. The movies constitute another excellent therapeutic measure for those who suffer in this way. Looked at in the proper way, they can be wonderfully restful and refreshing to eyes which react badly to the peculiar composition of fluorescent light and to minds which are baffled by the shadowless world of low contrasts in which that light compels them to work.

Appendix 1

In myopes especially, posture tends to be extremely bad. This may be directly due in some cases to the short sight, which encourages stooping and a hanging of the head. Conversely, the myopia may be due in part at least to the bad posture. F.M. Alexander records cases in which myopic children regained normal vision after being taught the proper way of carrying the head and neck in relation to the trunk.

In adults the correction of improper posture does not seem to be sufficient of itself to restore normal vision. Improvement in vision will be accelerated by those who learn to correct faulty habits of using the organism as a whole; but the simultaneous learning of the specific art of seeing is indispensable.

Design and illustrations by Michael Patrick Cronan
Typeset by Connie Wiggins